Clinical Manual for Treatment of Alcoholism and Addictions

Clinical Manual for Treatment of Alcoholism and Addictions

by

Avram H. Mack, M.D.

Attending Physician, Georgetown University Hospital, Washington, D.C.;
Associate Professor of Clinical Psychiatry, Georgetown University School
of Medicine, Washington, D.C.

Amy L. Harrington, M.D.

Physician, Georgetown University Hospital, Washington, D.C.

Richard J. Frances, M.D.

Clinical Professor of Psychiatry, New York University, New York City;
Adjunct Professor of Psychiatry, University of Medicine and Dentistry
of New Jersey, Newark, New Jersey;
and Director of Professional and Public Education,
Silver Hill Hospital, New Canaan, Connecticut

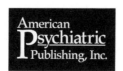

American Psychiatric Publishing, Inc.

Washington, DC
London, England

Books published by American Psychiatric Publishing, Inc., represent the views and opinions of the individual authors and do not necessarily represent the policies and opinions of APPI or the American Psychiatric Association.

If you would like to buy between 25 and 99 copies of this or any other APPI title, you are eligible for a 20% discount; please contact APPI Customer Service at appi@psych.org or 800-368-5777. If you wish to buy 100 or more copies of the same title, please e-mail us at bulksales@psych.org for a price quote.

Manufactured in the United States of America on acid-free paper
14   13   12   11   10   5   4   3   2   1
First Edition

Typeset in Adobe AGaramond and Formata.

American Psychiatric Publishing, Inc.
1000 Wilson Boulevard
Arlington, VA 22209-3901
www.appi.org

Library of Congress Cataloging-in-Publication Data
Mack, Avram H.
    Clinical manual for treatment of alcoholism and addictions / by Avram H. Mack, Amy L. Harrington, Richard J. Frances. — 1st ed.
        p. ; cm.
    Revision of: Concise guide to treatment of alcoholism and addictions / Avram H. Mack, John E. Franklin, Jr., Richard J. Frances. 2nd ed. c2001.
    Includes bibliographical references and index.
    ISBN 978-1-58562-373-0 (alk. paper)
    1. Substance abuse—Treatment—Handbooks, manuals, etc. 2. Alcoholism—Treatment—Handbooks, manuals, etc. I. Harrington, Amy L. II. Frances, Richard J. III. Mack, Avram H. Concise guide to treatment of alcoholism and addictions. IV. Title.
    [DNLM: 1. Substance-Related Disorders—therapy—Handbooks. 2. Behavior, Addictive—therapy—Handbooks.   WM 34 M153c 2010]
    RC564.F73 2010
    616.86′06—dc22
                                                                                            2009039467

British Library Cataloguing in Publication Data
A CIP record is available from the British Library.

Contents

Foreword

Substance use disorders are among the most complex and compromising health problems facing health care workers today. Up to 18% of Americans face a substance use problem some time during their lives. And federal, state, and local government spending on this public health problem is nearly half a trillion dollars each year (1). Fortunately, significant advances have been made in the treatment and underlying science of substance use disorders that enable clinicians to better treat substance abuse problems. The *Clinical Manual for Treatment of Alcoholism and Addictions* offers mental health workers in a variety of settings the clinically relevant information they need to address substance-related problems.

The *Clinical Manual for Treatment of Alcoholism and Addictions* is based on a revised edition of the *Concise Guide to Treatment of Alcoholism and Addictions*, now in a clinical manual format. This new clinical manual continues to provide easy-to-read and authoritative clinical information to guide health care professionals in the trenches with the latest clinical and research wisdom in a convenient form. The new manual format is larger, offers longer, more in-depth chapters, and allows for larger formatting of tables and figures. The manual provides practical advice clinicians can use every day.

Intended to complement *The American Psychiatric Publishing Textbook of Substance Abuse Treatment* (2) and other lengthier texts on the same subject, the *Clinical Manual for Treatment of Alcoholism and Addictions* is grounded in both the central importance of the doctor-patient relationship and in the empirically based DSM-IV-TR, systematically detailing all definitions and disorders within the addiction section.

The book also presents the latest research findings, including epidemiology data, treatment recommendations that address the newest medications and psychosocial therapeutic modalities. Its relevance is enhanced by the experience of all three authors, who treat addictions and their complications daily in both inpatient and outpatient clinical settings.

With its practical focus and broad range, this reference is useful for both students and practitioners. Although written for clinicians and other mental health care professionals, this guide will also be welcomed by allied professionals such as addiction counselors, lawyers, police and corrections officers, clergy, educators, and public policy makers.

More than 1,800 psychiatrists have been certified in addiction psychiatry. Unfortunately, however, less than half of the population in need of substance abuse treatment actually receives it. This is a function of both the reluctance of private and public payors to adequately fund treatment and the affected population to seek it. More needs to be done on this latter issue.

Drs. Mack, Harrington, and Frances have designed this volume to serve clinicians in practice as well as trainees in psychiatry who are concerned with addiction, general medicine, and other health professions. We believe that the book will serve as a valuable treatment resource for any health care professional concerned with the problems posed by patients with substance use disorders.

The *Clinical Manual for Treatment of Alcoholism and Addictions* is practical and clinically oriented. Research review and citations are kept to a minimum in favor of practical knowledge that readers can use in their everyday work with patients. Tables and figures provide easy access to large and complex pieces of information, and Key Clinical Points summarize the important take-away points for each chapter. Reference citations to the literature are limited; however, Suggested Readings are provided for each chapter for those interested in pursuing the topic further. Relevant Web sites are listed, where appropriate, for both clinicians and their patients. And representative case vignettes are used to enhance the clinical applicability of the information provided.

We believe this new manual will find a welcome place on the shelves of a wide variety of health care workers dealing with this devastating problem.

Marc Galanter, M.D.
Herbert D. Kleber, M.D.

References

1. News & Notes: Annual government spending on substance abuse and addiction nears a half trillion dollars. Psychiatr Serv 60:1000, 2009
2. Galanter M, Kleber HD (eds): The American Psychiatric Publishing Textbook of Substance Abuse Treatment, Fourth Edition. Washington, DC, 2008

Preface

In the United States, substance use disorders (SUDs) comprise a tremendous medical and social challenge: in 2007 19.9 million Americans were current users of illicit drugs, up from 14.8 million in 1999, and, including the related aspects of crime, absenteeism, and treatment, the monetary cost to the nation is estimated to be greater than $275 billion annually. Those in every category of health care—physicians, nurses, psychologists, social workers, alcohol and drug counselors, and rehabilitation therapists—and students in all of these areas are constantly faced with treatment choices and options that are critical to the care of patients with SUDs.

This manual is designed to be a concise guide containing useful tools for the treatment options offered by these professionals. Although primarily written with the clinician in mind, many allied helping professions such as the clergy, educators, lawyers, police officers, and corrections personnel will find the book useful. Education about addictions has been increasing recently for health professionals. Yet, considering the magnitude of the problem, this area remains underrepresented in the core of medical student and resident curricula, and both generalist and specialist training are needed for nurses, social workers, and psychologists. Addiction counselors need more psychiatric training to better deal with comorbidity.

This manual is an extensive revision of the second edition of our previous book, *Concise Guide to Treatment of Alcoholism and Addictions,* a concise overview of addiction treatment issues relevant to the clinician in the trenches and a distillation of our clinical experience as well as our review of the literature. The material in this manual has been improved by the suggestions of the readers of the concise guide.

During a 35-year period in the U.S. Navy, New York Hospital, New Jersey Medical School, Hackensack Hospital, and Silver Hill Hospital, Richard Frances, M.D., has had the opportunity to follow the treatment course and progress of 20,000–30,000 patients with SUDs and to supervise approximately 1,000 psychiatric residents, both individually and in their teams. As founding president of the American Academy of Addiction Psychiatry and as chair of the American Psychiatric Association Council on the Addictions, he has been a leader in the field, and helped establish ABPN Board Certification in Addiction Psychiatry as a subspecialty of psychiatry. At Cornell, the Harvard Longwood sites, Columbia-Presbyterian, Bellevue Hospital, Medical University of South Carolina, and Georgetown University Hospital, Avram H. Mack, M.D., has worked extensively with inpatient, outpatient, and consultation service treatment planning for this population, and has developed a special interest in child forensic issues. As a resident at Georgetown University Hospital and as a fellow in addiction psychiatry at Boston University, Amy L. Harrington, M.D., provides a fresh new perspective with a focus on the practical and educational needs of trainees.

The limitations of a handbook format, in terms of summarizing and highlighting the important issues, lead us to focus on what we believe to be the most important clinically relevant material, at the risk of omitting extensive presentations of research data and reviews of literature. We are grateful to Robert Hales, M.D., Carol Nadelson, M.D., John McDuffie, and Ron McMillen for their suggestions regarding the book; to our colleagues, staff, teachers, colleagues, and students, at New York Hospital-Cornell Medical Center, New Jersey Medical School, New York University Medical School, Silver Hill Hospital, Northwestern University Medical Center, Brigham and Women's Hospital, Massachusetts Mental Health Center, Beth Israel Deaconess Medical Center, Harvard Medical School, and Georgetown University Hospital, and to our patients, who have worked with us at understanding treatment problems. In addition, George Vaillant, M.D., John Renner, M.D., George Kolodner, M.D., Steven A. Epstein, M.D., Alan Newman, M.D., Hallie A. Lightdale, and Jeremy R. Mack, M.D., have provided invaluable support and guidance.

Avram H. Mack, M.D.
Amy L. Harrington, M.D.
Richard J. Frances, M.D.

1

Introduction

This guide to the treatment of substance use disorders (SUDs) disseminates information on the implications of new research on addiction treatment and a variety of approaches that have been useful to clinicians. Patients, their families, and clinicians face confusing choices about treatment combinations, which should be tailored to the individual. Data on optimal treatment combinations await valid and well-constructed outcome research. The current literature on SUD treatment outcomes is relatively nonspecific and of limited value in informing clinicians about the available tools that can be helpful. The clinician's choices are enhanced by obtaining a careful history and conducting thorough mental status and physical examination, as well as by using diagnostic formulations and confirmatory evidence from laboratory tests and third-party sources. The American Psychiatric Association practice guidelines on SUDs (Kleber et al. 2007) and the American Society of Addiction Medicine placement criteria (Mee-Lee et al. 2001) provide general principles for this developing field, as does the National Institute on Drug Abuse (2009) guide. The three institutes covering this field—National Institute on Mental Health, National Institute on Alcohol Abuse and Alcoholism, and National Institute on

1

Drug Abuse—have published an impressive array of educational and practice resources, most of which are available online. The current volume—representing the extensively updated and revised third edition of the *Concise Guide to Treatment of Alcoholism and Addictions* (now called *Clinical Manual for Treatment of Alcoholism and Addictions*)—was created for the clinician seeking practical, direct advice about common problems encountered in substance abuse treatment. In this chapter, we introduce some of the key issues in this increasingly complex field.

Treatment of SUDs can be extremely difficult. Helping to motivate the patient and family members to acknowledge the problem and to accept help are the two most important steps in treatment, recognized both by self-help groups and by research in motivational interviewing and stages of change (Prochaska et al. 1992). These steps are frequently difficult because of the nature of addictive disorders, which leads to denial, lying, and organicity. Both patient and therapist may struggle with the stigma of SUDs and with accepting that the patient has an illness. With this illness comes the personal responsibility of the patient to acknowledge that he or she needs help and to cooperate with a treatment plan. Most often, a patient will prefer to have a goal of controlled use and will initially have difficulty accepting a therapist's standard of abstinence as the goal for treatment. A patient will frequently feel hopeless about ever achieving sustained abstinence and may need to be encouraged that this goal is attainable. Seeing others who are recovering and personally experiencing increasing periods of abstinence will help bolster hope.

Self-efficacy is a capacity that should be fostered by the clinician. It refers to the patient's capacity to take control of his or her life; to improve self-care; and to make decisions, such as that of becoming sober and clean. This quality is an important prognostic sign and an ingredient of any recovery, and helps improve self-esteem and coping skills.

The clinician makes efforts to prevent lapses from turning into relapses by encouraging honesty, by openly providing support, and by encouraging a quick return to treatment. Discussing and weighing the pros and cons of continuing his or her current addiction-driven lifestyle with the patient are important in helping shift the decisional balance to strengthen motivation for and efforts at recovery. The full benefits of a healthy lifestyle and what the patient has to gain from sobriety are as important as helping the patient face the full impact and impairment of his or her untreated addiction. Harm avoidance approaches such as needle exchange, relapse prevention, and maintenance treatment with pharmacological and psychotherapeutic modalities for patients with comorbidity can be combined with a long-range goal of abstinence. Unfortunately, the term *harm avoidance* is also sometimes used as part of the justification for legalization of illicit substances, a position we oppose. Legalization would increase availability and lower costs of drugs, and it would increase the number of complications and the comorbidity of SUDs. Prevention and treatment should be made more widely available to reduce use; and drug courts and mental health courts are viable alternatives to the traditional criminal justice system. More treatment, including detoxification, should be available to prisoners as well (and in a timely fashion—see Chapter 7, "Violence and Suicide, Injury, Corrections, and Forensics," in this manual). Drug substitution (for example, methadone or buprenorphine maintenance) and the use of other indicated medications may be met with resistance that will often need to be worked through.

Treatment of Substance Use Disorders: General Tenets

Below we introduce some of the key tenets of substance abuse treatment:

1. *Case heterogeneity.* The patient is an individual and varies in terms of substance(s) used, pattern of use, severity of abuse or dependence, degree of functional impairment, secondary medical conditions, psychiatric comorbidity, strengths and vulnerabilities, and social and environmental context. Thus, no one treatment works for all individuals.
2. *Phases of treatment.* Active treatment progresses: it does not all happen at once. The clinician should begin with comprehensive assessment and move to treatment of intoxication or withdrawal, development of a treatment plan, and enactment of the plan. The patient is initially in the action phase (which lasts approximately 6 months) and then moves on to the maintenance phase of sobriety. The amount of time spent in treatment is a critical prognostic factor.
3. *Comprehensive assessment and treatment.* Both assessment and treatment must take into account all aspects of the individual's life and illness. Col-

lateral sources of information are extremely important in assessment. Co-existing psychiatric and medical conditions should be treated concurrently in an integrated manner. Treatment programs should assess for human immunodeficiency virus (HIV), hepatitis, tuberculosis, and other infectious diseases and should provide education to help patients reduce their risk of contracting communicable diseases.

4. *Treatment planning.* Goals of treatment should include reduction of substance use, achievement of abstinence, diminishment of relapse frequency, and enhancement of rehabilitation and recovery. Treatment status must be continually reviewed, reassessed, and updated.

5. *Perspectives on relapse.* Although not desirable, relapses do occur; all treatment plans must assess for them. Relapses do not always imply treatment failure; treatment continues. Relapse triggers must be identified, coping skills enhanced, and treatment of comorbid conditions reassessed; efforts must be made to motivate the patient to get back on track, with increased surveillance in place as appropriate. Abstinence may sometimes seem an impossible goal (e.g., in elderly patients), but reductions in morbidity and mortality follow any decreases in substance use, making the effort worthwhile (Marlatt and Gordon 1985).

6. *Stages of change.* A central paradigm developed by Prochaska et al. (1992) defined a continuum of phases ("stages") through which an addicted individual passes on the road to recovery: precontemplation, contemplation, action, preparation, and maintenance. The *stages of change* model can be applied to a variety of illnesses, including addiction. It can be very useful in treatment planning: by tailoring treatment interventions to the patient's specific stage in the recovery process, the clinician can help the patient to progress through the continuum toward health.

7. *Craving.* Craving can be a factor leading to relapse. The patient should be reminded that craving is to be expected, is time-limited, and (unlike hunger or the need to urinate) can fluctuate, fade, or disappear over time. Medications such as naltrexone and disulfiram reduce craving for alcohol after detoxification, and appropriate medications to attenuate withdrawal symptoms are also helpful. Once the idea of "no drinking, no drugging, no matter what" becomes part of the patient's lifestyle, it removes the acceptability of the choice of using, thereby indirectly reducing craving.

Therapeutic Alliance

The therapeutic alliance may be one of the clinician's most important tools. Having frequently grown up in families with SUDs, it is not surprising that the patient with a substance abuse problem is likely to have typical transference resistances to treatment and is likely to evoke countertransference reactions in the therapist that may either facilitate or undermine treatment, depending on how the reactions are handled (Frances 1998). Therapists who are well informed and well trained and who understand and are in touch with their own feelings are more helpful to patients and are less likely to experience "burnout" (Frances and Alexopoulos 1982). We offer 10 therapist attributes and attitudes that are helpful in working with patients with SUDs:

1. The most crucial nonspecific variable is an attitude of respect for the provision of a caring and compassionate relationship. Often underestimated, a concern for the patient and a willingness to form an active therapeutic alliance (with some degree of therapeutic zeal, but without overidentification) are critical for work with patients who have SUDs. An empathic capacity to feel the patient's experience, yet maintain objectivity, is crucial. Following a psychotherapeutic tradition of activity (which goes back to Ferenczi and Alexander), the therapist takes an active role in creating an environment in which the patient can achieve comfort and growth. The therapist's ability to confront with concern as well as provide emotional support appropriately are desirable attributes. This does not mean playing a real parental role or taking a contrived position that is not genuinely felt by the therapist. It is important that the therapist not abuse the power that the patient invests in him or her, but rather exercise it with decency and compassion.

2. The therapist should be an informed optimist. It has been said that the difference between an optimist and a pessimist is that the pessimist is better informed. However, therapeutic nihilism or overidentification with a patient's helplessness, low self-esteem, and hopelessness often contributes to poor treatment results. An informed optimism based on one's experience of having helped patients, knowledge of the course and treatment of addictions, and memories of working with patients who have done well is a tremendous asset to any therapist. The clinician should have zeal and

be an activist in fostering the patient's successful recovery. Every day sober is an achievement! Acceptance of the limits of treatment and of the chronic nature of SUDs, however, is equally important.

3. The therapist's capacity to tolerate anxiety, pain, frustration, and depression is essential. When therapists are unaware of their own weaknesses and sensitive areas, they may find themselves colluding with patients in avoiding painful areas. By contrast, therapists who acknowledge, face, and explore painful topics provide patients with a valuable alternative model for dealing with negative affects without resorting to substance use. Therapists who know themselves and can tolerate depression are also able to work with more difficult cases.

4. Flexibility and open-mindedness are desirable therapist traits. Simple answers to complicated problems, applied uniformly, without taking into account special circumstances, are often wrong. Dogmatically held positions by therapists and treatment programs may lead to blind spots, facilitate splitting, and recreate an atmosphere of conflict already familiar in patients' lives. Flexibility can involve bringing together several modalities of treatment, trying a sequence of different modalities to see what works best, and being willing to seek consultation and supervision in difficult cases. The kind of flexibility discussed here is entirely compatible with setting strict limits and providing a consistency of approach.

5. In addition to a strong knowledge of general psychiatry, resourcefulness, creativity, and familiarity with numerous treatment modalities are extremely helpful characteristics for the therapist.

6. Intellectual curiosity is vital to the therapist's growth. It is essential that the therapist keep up with the clinical and research literature. The therapist should have an active interest and curiosity in learning more about the needs of each patient.

7. The best therapists possess wisdom. This may grow with the therapist's work and life experience and is enhanced by humility and a sense of humor. Many fine therapists are able to use metaphors in ways that capture images of immense usefulness to their patients. For example, the eminent behavioral psychologist Howard Hunt once told an acting-out polysubstance abuser that he was behaving like a loose cannon on the deck of a rolling wooden ship in a storm. On another occasion, Hunt compared a self-defeating alcoholic patient to a child who is always reaching for ice

cream cones only to have them melt before they reach his lips. Perhaps wisdom is best stated in the Serenity Prayer, which seeks "the serenity to accept the things I cannot change, the courage to change the things I can, and the wisdom to know the difference."

8. Persistence and patience are qualities that are as valuable to clinicians as they are to researchers. Like a fisherman chasing a marlin, the therapist must be able to wait, work hard, and be prepared for either little or late ultimate gratification from a case.

9. The capacity to listen and to hear both what is and what is not said and to act accordingly is very important. This includes sharing with the patient what has been heard, as well as attending to negative responses from patients—"You listen but you don't hear"; "You don't listen"; "You aren't seeing what I am really like." These statements may be accurate, or they may represent the way the patient felt about parents or other figures in the patient's life. Given the propensity for denial in this population, the clinician must be vigilant for signs and symptoms of problems. In the SUD field, because of the emphasis on psychoeducation and counseling, the basic skills of listening must always be emphasized.

10. Honesty and integrity in the therapist and in the treatment team are crucial. Extremely sensitive to deception and frequently mistrustful, the patient will need to have an ongoing, consistent experience with a therapist worthy of trust. In working with patients with SUDs who have experienced a regression or erosion of their value systems, examination of values almost inevitably becomes part of treatment. The therapist's integrity is an important asset in this exploration. Common and sometimes subtle forms of corruption of the treatment can occur and must be carefully avoided. The team approach can frequently lead to an open and honest discussion, which may help individuals face their own countertransference issues and strengthen the overall treatment.

Potential Abuses in the Treatment of Substance Use Disorders

Table 1–1 presents examples of more or less subtle forms of corruption that individual therapists and treatment programs must attempt to avoid and seek to manage if they occur.

Table 1–1. Potential abuses in the treatment of substance use disorders

Preferential treatment influenced by VIP pressures, resulting in mistakes and splitting in the team

Distortions of diagnosis (e.g., underdiagnosis of alcoholism because of fears or pressure)

Premature discharge to save money

Ordering of excessive laboratory tests or diagnostic measures and overcharging for services

Excessively punitive or critical approaches, with constant threats of discharge in patients who are resistant to treatment

Breaches of confidentiality, leading to major problems in trust

Key Points

- Treatment of SUDs requires the consistent application of fundamental clinical skills.
- Clinicians should expect cravings and relapses in the substance-dependent population.
- Clinicians need to be aware of potential pitfalls in the therapeutic relationship in addiction practice.

References

Frances RJ: Addiction treatment: avoiding pitfalls—a case approach. An overview. Group for Advancement of Psychiatry (GAP Report 142). Washington, DC, American Psychiatric Press 142:1–9, 1998

Frances RJ, Alexopoulos GS: Patient management and education: getting the alcoholic into treatment. Physician and Patient 1(6):9–14, 1982

Kleber HD, Weiss RD, Anton RF Jr, et al: Treatment of patients with substance use disorders, second edition. Work Group on Substance Use Disorders; American Psychiatric Association; Steering Committee on Practice Guidelines. Am J Psychiatry 164 (4 suppl):5–123, 2007

Marlatt GA, Gordon JR: Relapse Prevention: Maintenance Strategies in the Treatment of Addictive Behaviors. New York, Guilford, 1985

Mee-Lee D, Shulman GR, Fishman M, et al: ASAM PPC-2R: American Society of Addiction Medicine Patient Placement Criteria for the Treatment of Substance-Related Disorders, 2nd Edition—Revised. Chevy Chase, MD, American Society of Addiction Medicine, 2001

National Institute on Drug Abuse: Principles of Drug Addiction Treatment: A Research-Based Guide, 2nd Edition (NIH Publ No 09-4180). Bethesda, MD, U.S. Department of Health and Human Services, April 2009

Prochaska JO, DiClemente CC, Norcross JC: In search of how people change: applications to addictive behavior. Am Psychol 47:1102–1114, 1992

2

Magnitude of the Problem

General Epidemiology

Substance use disorders (SUDs) are likely the most prevalent of all types of medical and mental disorders, and they cost society greatly. In this chapter, we focus on the epidemiology of SUDs. We have gathered most of our data from numerous studies: the Drug Abuse Warning Network (DAWN; Substance Abuse and Mental Health Services Administration 2008a), which provides ongoing surveillance data on emergency department visits and deaths due to substance misuse; the Monitoring the Future study, an ongoing study of substance abuse among American high school and college students and young adults (Johnston et al. 2008); the National Survey on Drug Use and Health (formerly called the National Household Survey; Substance Abuse and Mental Health Services Administration 2008b); findings from the Epidemiologic Catchment Area (ECA) Study, which have been updated in specific areas regarding substances (Regier et al. 1990); and the National Comorbidity Survey Replication (NCS-R; Kessler et al. 2005).

11

Facts of General Magnitude

We begin with an overview of use of substances generally.

- In 2007, 19.9 million Americans were current users of illicit drugs, up from 14.8 million in 1999 (Substance Abuse and Mental Health Services Administration 2008b).
- Between 2002 and 2007, the number of persons meeting diagnostic criteria for substance abuse or dependence remained relatively stable, at around 22.0 million (Substance Abuse and Mental Health Services Administration 2008b).
- Between 2003 and 2004, drug abuse deaths reported to DAWN increased in most states and in most metropolitan areas (Substance Abuse and Mental Health Services Administration 2008a).
- Current illicit drug use among persons ages 12–17 years continued to trend downward, from 11.6% in 2002 to 9.5% in 2007. The rate was highest (16.3%) in 1979 and lowest (5.3%) in 1992. The age group with the highest prevalence of drug use (19.7%) was young adults ages 18–25 years (Substance Abuse and Mental Health Services Administration 2008b).
- Drug use among persons ages 50–59 years has been rising, possibly reflecting the aging of the Baby Boomers. Between 2002 and 2006, the rate of drug use increased from 3.4% to 6.0%, then held steady at 5.7% in 2007. Between 2002 and 2007, drug use among persons ages 55–59 years increased from 1.9% to 4.1%.
- In 2007, 1.6% of the population and 57.4% of those with an SUD used marijuana, making it the drug with the highest rate of abuse or dependence in that year (Substance Abuse and Mental Health Services Administration 2008b).
- According to DAWN estimates, more than 1.7 million of the 113 million emergency department visits in 2006 were associated with drug misuse or abuse. Of these, 958,164 (55%) involved an illicit drug. Approximately 57% involved cocaine, 30% involved marijuana, 19% involved heroin, and 11% involved stimulants and amphetamines. Other illicit drugs reported to DAWN included 3,4-methylenedioxymethamphetamine (MDMA, Ecstasy), phencyclidine (PCP), lysergic acid diethylamide

(LSD), gamma-hydroxybutyrate (GHB), and miscellaneous hallucinogens (Substance Abuse and Mental Health Services Administration 2008a).

* Regarding youth perceptions of the risk and availability of drugs, between 2002 and 2007 there was a slight increase in the proportion of youth ages 12–17 years who perceived "great risk" from marijuana use (32.4% to 34.5%) or from binge drinking (38.2% to 39.4%). On the other hand, the proportion of youth who thought that trying heroin once or twice was a great risk decreased from 58.5% to 57.0%, and the percentage of those who thought that trying LSD once or twice was a great risk decreased from 52.6% to 51.6%. The percentage of youth who felt that using cocaine once or twice a month was a great risk stayed relatively stable between 2002 and 2007, at roughly 50% (Substance Abuse and Mental Health Services Administration 2008b).

Societal Cost

With their vast impact on our culture and society, SUDs may well become the main challenge for psychiatry and society in the twenty-first century. In addition to representing a primary public health problem, SUDs greatly affect the economic, political, and social fabric of the nation, play a role in international relations, and fund various nefarious international organizations. Measures of the problem include per capita consumption, lifetime and point prevalence, morbidity and mortality, fetal effects of drugs, health care costs, and total costs of lost worktime. Not only do drug and alcohol abuse lead to higher health care costs for addicted persons, but they also affect the families of people abusing drugs and alcohol. Children of parents who abuse drugs and alcohol are at increased risk with regard to their health, their school performance, and their chances of abusing drugs and alcohol themselves, and these children are often in need of long-term supportive services (Regier et al. 1990). The actual monetary cost to the nation is estimated to be greater than $500 billion annually, including the related aspects of crime, absenteeism, and treatment (Harwood 2000). Also, 30%–55% of mentally ill persons have an SUD, multiplying the cost of treating primary mental illness (Kessler et al. 1997).

Substances of Abuse and Misuse

Alcohol

This section reviews the epidemiology of alcohol use specifically.

- In 2007, the lifetime prevalence of alcohol abuse, with or without dependence, was 13.2%; 3.1% had met criteria for alcohol abuse in the previous 12 months (Substance Abuse and Mental Health Services Administration 2008b).
- The most reliable estimate of the annual cost attributed to alcohol is $191.6 billion, almost double that of the late 1980s (Harwood 2000).
- A review of 15,495 violent deaths in 2005 revealed that 59.1% of the decedents had blood alcohol levels greater than 0.08. This included 62.1% of suicide decedents with a blood alcohol level greater than the legal limit in most states (Karch et al. 2008).
- In 2006, 32% of all driving fatalities were related to excessive alcohol use (National Highway Traffic Safety Administration 2008).
- In 2005, 33.9% of eighth graders, 56.7% of tenth graders, and 68.6% of twelfth graders reported using alcohol in the past year. This represented a drop of 2.7%, 1.5%, and 2.1% respectively. The percentage of eighth, tenth, and twelfth graders who binge drank or drank more than 5 alcoholic beverages in 1 day in the past month was 17%, 33%, and 47%, respectively (Johnston et al. 2008).

Morbidity and mortality secondary to alcohol depend on the culture to which the user belongs. The average American over age 14 years consumes 2.77 gallons of absolute alcohol annually, which is less than in Russia, France, Scandinavia, and Ireland but more than in Islamic and Mediterranean cultures or China. In the United States, approximately one-tenth of those who drink consume half the alcohol sold.

Alcohol's public health effects are tremendous. The suicide rate in persons with alcoholism without any comorbid conditions is about 5%–6%, much higher than that in the general population. Alcoholism is the leading associated factor for cirrhosis, even though fewer than 10% of alcoholics develop cirrhosis. There is a high association between alcohol and/or drug use and violent crime and accidents. About 25% of people admitted to general hospitals have problems related to chronic alcohol use (e.g., cirrhosis, cardiomyopathy) or problems related to withdrawal (e.g., seizures, pneumonia, liver failure, subdural hematomas).

Cocaine

This section reviews the epidemiology of cocaine use specifically.

- In 2007, an estimated 2.1 million Americans were current cocaine users (Substance Abuse and Mental Health Services Administration 2008b).
- In 2007, there were 906,000 people over age 12 years who used cocaine for the first time in the preceding 12 months. And 66.5% of recent cocaine initiates were age 18 years or older at first use (Substance Abuse and Mental Health Services Administration 2008b).
- In 2003, 9.4% of those who completed suicide tested positive for cocaine at autopsy (Karch et al. 2008).
- In 2007, approximately 2,500 people per day, or 906,000 people in total, used cocaine for the first time. The average age at first use has remained steady in recent years, at roughly 20.2 years (Substance Abuse and Mental Health Services Administration 2008b).

Although the epidemic use of cocaine in the 1980s abated around 1990, a significant increase in use occurred from 1991 to 1997. In 2007, cocaine was the illicit drug with the third-highest level of past-year dependence or abuse (1.6 million), following only marijuana use (3.9 million) and pain reliever misuse (1.7 million) (Substance Abuse and Mental Health Services Administration 2008b). Increased marketing pressures, lower prices, and availability of more potent, fast-acting cocaine derivatives that can be smoked or used intravenously (e.g., "crack") have increased experimentation, availability, and prevalence of dependence. Interestingly, in the 1970s, experimentation with cocaine was considered relatively safe by many young people and was thought by some experts to not be very dangerous. Cocaine psychosis was rarely reported; lower dosages of cocaine were used, and reports of major complications were rare. This happened to coincide with a period of time during which use of cocaine was increasing. Since the 1980s, increased market demand has been accompanied by increased availability of purer, more potent forms at lower prices, with more rapid routes of administration, contributing to more frequent severe complications, shortening ("telescoping") of the progression from use to addiction, and wider problems across social class and race. After the cocaine-related death of Len Bias, a first-round NBA draft pick from the University of Maryland at the end of his senior year of college in 1986, perceived risk of cocaine use steadily increased and use decreased. Since the late 1990s, perceived risk of cocaine use has leveled off to about 55% among eighth, tenth, and twelfth graders (Johnston et al. 2008). Disapproval of ever trying crack cocaine is slightly higher but has also leveled off over the past several years (Johnston et al. 2008).

Amphetamines

This section reviews the epidemiology of amphetamine (including methamphetamine) use specifically.

- Annual prevalence rates for use of methamphetamine among eighth, tenth, and twelfth graders in 2008 were 12%, 15%, and 12%, respectively. While any such use is alarming, these figures are down from rates of 32%, 46%, and 47%, respectively, in 1999 (Johnston et al. 2008).
- The number of people who use methamphetamine has declined slightly, from 1.9 million (0.8%) in 2006 to 1.3 million (0.5%) in 2007 (Substance Abuse and Mental Health Services Administration 2008b).
- Drug abuse–related emergency department visits involving amphetamines increased 54% between 1995 and 2002 (from 25,245 to 38,961 emergency department visits) (Substance Abuse and Mental Health Services Administration 2004b).
- Emergency department visits related to methamphetamine peaked at 132,576 in 2004 but declined to 109,655 and 79,924 in 2005 and 2006, respectively (Substance Abuse and Mental Health Services Administration 2008b).
- The number of recent new users of methamphetamine was significantly lower in 2007 than in 2002. Past-year initiates of methamphetamine dropped from 299,000 in 2002 to 157,000 in 2007, with a peak use of 318,000 in 2004 (Substance Abuse and Mental Health Services Administration 2008a).

The diversion and abuse of amphetamines, which are often prescribed in the treatment of narcolepsy, weight disorders, and depressive disorders, peaked in the 1960s. With better control, legal use, diversion, and illegal use declined. Unfortunately, methamphetamine can be synthesized using household supplies and over-the-counter medications. This process can produce toxic waste products and can cause explosions. There have been attempts in recent years to curb access to the medicines that serve as precursors to methamphetamine by limiting the quantity that can be sold to one person and restricting the sale of these medications to persons older than 17 years.

Opioids

This section reviews the epidemiology of opioid use specifically.

- Lifetime heroin use prevalence estimates have ranged from 2.3 million in 1979 to 1.7 million in 1992, 2 million in 1997, 2.4 million in 1998, and more than 3.7 million in 2007 and 2008 (Substance Abuse and Mental Health Services Administration 2009b).
- An estimated 114,000 persons used heroin for the first time in 2008, which was not statistically significantly different from the 117,000 initiates in 2002 but which differed greatly from the 149,000 in 1999.
- The estimated number of current heroin users was 68,000 in 1993, 117,000 in 1994, 196,000 in 1995, 216,000 in 1996, 325,000 in 1997, 130,000 in 1998, 200,000 in 1999, and 213,000 in 2008 (Substance Abuse and Mental Health Services Administration 2009b).
- The DAWN study revealed that emergency department visits associated with misuse or abuse of opiates/opioids increased 24% from 2004 to 2005, and visits associated with methadone increased 29% (Substance Abuse and Mental Health Services Administration 2008a).
- Nearly one-third of the 2.7 million people who used illicit drugs for the first time in 2007 initiated with prescription pain relievers, making these agents second only to marijuana in terms of reported first drugs (Substance Abuse and Mental Health Services Administration 2008b). Prescription pain medication misuse increased among young adults (ages 18–25 years) between 2002 and 2007, from 4.1% to 4.6% (Substance Abuse and Mental Health Services Administration 2009b).

- The number of new nonmedical users of oxycodone was 554,000 in 2007, with an average age of first use of 24 years (Substance Abuse and Mental Health Services Administration 2008b).

It is difficult to obtain accurate data on opioid use; estimates come from overdose reports, surveys, prevalence of medical complications, arrests, and treatment program admissions. Heroin abuse is usually a problem among urban males and in the 18- to 25-year age group. Increasing evidence suggests that misuse of prescription opiates is a growing problem and is affecting new populations that had previously avoided the heroin epidemic. There have been several highly publicized deaths of celebrities in recent years in which misuse of opioids, in particular methadone, has been implicated. Emergency department visits related specifically to opiate use increased at a rate 10 times that of the rate of increase of emergency department visits in general.

In addition to lacking adequate availability of treatment openings, most methadone programs lack the capacity for intensive treatment, including enough individual and group counseling, a team approach, and the increasingly important medical and psychiatric support. Unfortunately, most people with psychoactive SUDs, including narcotics addicts, are not in treatment. As more physicians become trained and certified in the prescription of buprenorphine for the treatment of opiate addiction, there are greater possibilities for reaching patients in order to treat them (Substance Abuse and Mental Health Services Administration 2004a). Insurance parity for mental health that includes addictions can also improve access to care. Providing addiction treatment access to the uninsured should be a priority for health care reform.

According to the DAWN report "Narcotic Analgesics, 2002 Update" (Substance Abuse and Mental Health Services Administration 2004c), the incidence of abuse of prescription opioid pain medications such as hydrocodone, oxycodone, meperidine, and propoxyphene has risen markedly in recent years. The incidence of emergency department visits related to these medications has been increasing since the 1990s and more than doubled between 1994 and 2001 (Substance Abuse and Mental Health Services Administration 2008a). In 2001 there were an estimated 90,232 emergency department visits related to opioid analgesic abuse, a 117% increase since 1994. Nationally, opioid analgesics were involved in 14% of all drug abuse–related emergency department visits in 2001 (Substance Abuse and Mental

Health Services Administration 2008a). According to *Mortality Data From the Drug Abuse Warning Network, 2002* (Substance Abuse and Mental Health Services Administration 2004d), hydrocodone ranked among the 10 most common drugs related to deaths (as certified by coroner) in a sample of 18 cities, including Detroit (63 hydrocodone-induced deaths), Las Vegas (46), Dallas (36), New Orleans (33), and Oklahoma City (31). Oxycodone ranked among the 10 most common drugs related to deaths in a sample of 19 cities, including Philadelphia (88 oxycodone-induced deaths), Baltimore (34), Boston (34), Phoenix (34), and Miami (28).

Tobacco

This section reviews the epidemiology of tobacco use specifically.

- In 2007, 28.6% of Americans age 12 years or older were current users of tobacco products. This included 24.2% of the population who smoked cigarettes, 5.4% who smoked cigars, 3.2% who used smokeless tobacco, and 0.8% who smoked tobacco in pipes (Substance Abuse and Mental Health Services Administration 2008b).
- In 2007, reported past-month use of any tobacco product was 12.4% in the 12- to 17-year age group, correlating to roughly 3.1 million adolescents. Of those, 2.5 million (9.8%) had used cigarettes and 1.1 million (4.2%) had used cigars. Smokeless tobacco use in this age group was up, from 2.0% in 2002 to 2.4% in 2007 (Johnston et al. 2008).
- In 2007, reported past-month smoking was 18.9% among youth ages 16–17 years and 8.4% among those ages 14–15 years. The peak age range for cigarette use was 38.5% among young adults ages 21–25 years. This was down from 40.2% for the same age group in 2006 and down from 41.6% in 1998, though up from 34.6% in 1994 (Substance Abuse and Mental Health Services Administration 2009b).
- In terms of race and ethnicity, prevalence of past-month smoking in 2007 was greater among American Indians/Alaska Natives (41.8%) and non-Hispanic whites (30.7%) than most other groups, including non-Hispanic blacks (26.8%), Hispanics (22.7%), or Asians/Pacific Islanders (15.4%) (Substance Abuse and Mental Health Services Administration 2009b).

- With regard to education and socioeconomic status, current smoking was highest among persons who had not graduated from high school (32.9%) and least among those who were college graduates (14.0%). It was higher for persons who were unemployed (44.6%) than it was for people who were working full-time (27.6%) or part-time (24.5%) (Substance Abuse and Mental Health Services Administration 2008b).

In general, use of tobacco products has decreased in the past decades. Educational campaigns, self-help groups, self-help literature, treatment facilities, and government legislation have been aimed at decreasing the numbers of smokers. Smoking in public places (e.g., restaurants, airplanes, hospitals, and work environments) is increasingly restricted and the rights of nonsmokers are being considered. In many cities, such as Boston and New York, smoking bans have been in place for many years. Restaurant and bars in these cities are seeing that the bans have not had the negative financial effects that opponents of the bans had predicted.

Hallucinogens and Club Drugs

This section reviews the epidemiology of hallucinogen and "club drug" use specifically.

- Among people using an illicit substance for the first time in 2007, 2.0% used a hallucinogen (Substance Abuse and Mental Health Services Administration 2008b).
- In 2007, 0.8 million people used Ecstasy for the first time and 0.3 million people used LSD for the first time (Substance Abuse and Mental Health Services Administration 2008b).
- The rate of current use of hallucinogens was 0.4% in 2007, which was the same rate of use reported in 1999. MDMA accounted for approximately half of this use (Substance Abuse and Mental Health Services Administration 2008b).

LSD achieved its greatest popularity in the 1960s and 1970s but has once again become popular in some high school communities. Some students have discovered that LSD is not easily detectable in urine samples. In the 1960s, psychedelic drugs were romanticized as part of a cultural movement that included a style of mind expansion and poetic expression in rock culture, and they became associated with turning away from war, rebelling against society, and "dropping out." Southwest American Indians had long used psilocybin in religious ceremonies. Although there have been few new drugs in the indolealkylamine derivatives category (which includes LSD), there has been a steady flow of new "designer" phenylalkylamine derivatives, including ring-substituted amphetamines such as 3,4-methylenedioxyamphetamine (MDA; "old Ecstasy"), MDMA ("new Ecstasy"), and 3,4-methylenedioxy-*N*-ethyl-amphetamine (MDEA). Ecstasy first appeared at "raves" but has grown in popularity and is increasingly implicated in deaths. There are 12 known natural hallucinogens and more than 100 synthetics to date. Other drugs that are seen at raves and are sometimes referred to as "club drugs" include ketamine, GHB, flunitrazepam (Rohypnol), and PCP. PCP ("angel dust") abuse is frequently associated with violent and bizarre behavior. PCP use had reached a nadir in the 1990s but in recent years has become popular again. Ketamine use has also risen in the past few years.

Cannabis

This section reviews the epidemiology of cannabis use specifically.

- Of the 2.7 million people who used illicit drugs for the first time in 2007, over one-half (56.2%) used marijuana as their first drug (Substance Abuse and Mental Health Services Administration 2008b).
- In 2007, 3.6 million people were using marijuana on a daily or an almost daily basis (more than 300 days in 1 year). Of those who had used the drug in the prior 30 days, over one-third, 5.1 million, had used marijuana for 20 or more of those days (Substance Abuse and Mental Health Services Administration 2008b).
- In 2007, there were roughly 6,000 new marijuana users a day. This figure has remained relatively stable since 2002 (Substance Abuse and Mental Health Services Administration 2008b).
- In 2007, males age 12 years or older were twice as likely to have used marijuana in the past 30 days as females (Substance Abuse and Mental Health Services Administration 2008b).

- The prevalence of current marijuana use among male youth declined from 9.1% in 2002 to 6.8% in 2007. For female youth, the rate of current marijuana use decreased from 7.2% in 2002 to 5.8% in 2007 (Substance Abuse and Mental Health Services Administration 2008b).

Worldwide, cannabis may be the most widely abused illicit substance of all; in the United States, it accounts for 75% of all illicit drug use. Trends and demographic characteristics for marijuana/hashish use are generally similar to those for other illicit drug use. Greater cannabis potency and heavier use have led to increased medical and psychological risks. Marijuana use peaked among adolescents in the 1970s; however, it continues to be a gateway drug for other substances of abuse. The perception of risk among adolescents remained stable from 2003 to 2007 (Substance Abuse and Mental Health Services Administration 2009a), which is a concern.

Inhalants

This section reviews the epidemiology of inhalant use specifically.

- In 2007, 775,000 people age 12 years or older used inhalants for the first time. The average age at first use increased from 15.7 years in 2006 to 17.1 in 2007 (Substance Abuse and Mental Health Services Administration 2008b).
- In 2003, 12.1% of students ages 12–17 reported using inhalants at any point in their lifetime. The past-month prevalence of inhalant use was 3.9% (Johnston et al. 2008).
- In 2003, there was a statistically significant 1.0-point increase in use by eighth graders, and in 2004 there were significant increases in inhalant use by eighth, tenth, and twelfth graders (Johnston et al. 2008).

Inhalant use stabilized in 1996 after 4 years of increase, according to the National High School Senior and Young Adult Survey (Johnston et al. 1997). The trend noted in the Monitoring the Future study demonstrating increased inhalant use in eighth, tenth, and twelfth grade students halted in 2005 for the younger grades, but use continued to increase for twelfth graders (Johnston et al. 2008). This, in combination with the increase in mean age at first use, could be an indicator that inhalant use by adults is a trend to watch.

Sedatives, Hypnotics, and Anxiolytics

This section reviews the epidemiology of sedative, hypnotic, and anxiolytic use specifically.

- In 2007, reported past-month use of tranquilizers and sedatives was 0.7% and 0.1%, respectively, and use remained fairly steady between 2002 and 2007 (Substance Abuse and Mental Health Services Administration 2008b).

- Emergency department visits related to nonmedical use of benzodiazepines increased 19% in 2005 (Substance Abuse and Mental Health Services Administration 2008a).

- Use of benzodiazepines among twelfth graders steadily increased from 1992 until roughly 2002–2005. In 2005, the annual prevalence of barbiturate use by twelfth graders was 7.2% (Johnston et al. 2008).

Although use of benzodiazepines and sedatives steadily declined during the 1980s and 1990s, there has been a recent trend toward increased use, particularly among teenagers. Abuse of these agents is related to the high prevalence of anxiety disorders. Barbiturate overdoses, once frequently the cause of emergency department visits, have declined because of the decreasing popularity of barbiturate prescription and use. They have been replaced by benzodiazepines, which have a higher index of therapeutic safety and a lower risk of causing respiratory depression.

Physicians prescribing benzodiazepines need to be aware of these agents' potential for abuse, especially by individuals with risk factors for alcohol and drug problems. It is difficult to get a coherent picture of the incidence and prevalence of alcoholism and other drug abuse because of a lack of clear criteria for diagnosis of dependence, variations of subpopulations studied, tolerance of a particular subculture for drug-related behaviors, and dishonesty in reporting of substance problems. It is important that physicians be aware of the potential for tolerance with these medications and to taper them gradually rather than abruptly discontinue them.

Prescription Medicine Misuse

A wide range of medications prescribed for typical medical or surgical conditions are increasingly being misused, a trend that has drawn a great deal of attention from government and professional institutions. Of particular concern is the stealing or taking of these medications by others in a household.

Polysubstance Problems

This section reviews the epidemiology of polysubstance use specifically.

- In the ECA Study, 30% of alcoholics also met criteria for abuse of or dependence on other substances (Regier et al. 1990).
- In the ECA Study, the most common comorbidity with an SUD was another SUD, nicotine dependence—which may have effects on treatment of a patient's psychiatric conditions and/or extrapyramidal side effects (Regier et al. 1990).
- In the ECA Study data, calculated odds ratios for SUDs among populations with specific disorders were as follows: major depressive disorder: 2, panic disorder: 3, schizophrenia: 5, and bipolar disorder: 7 (Regier et al. 1990).

Recently, polysubstance abuse has increased, with combined use of alcohol, heroin, cocaine, methadone, and tobacco. Use of combinations of substances has been especially noted in young and female patients. Teenagers tend to progress from alcohol and tobacco use to marijuana use and use of barbiturates, codeine, or other opioids before abusing heroin. Deaths related to overdose are more commonly associated with combinations of alcohol, depressants, and heroin than with cocaine, which has recently received greater public attention. Of note, treatment for abuse of one substance usually has the effect of reducing use of others (e.g., a methadone maintenance program reduces comorbid cocaine abuse).

Underlying Issues Affecting Addiction Magnitude

Medical and Psychiatric Complications

Medical and psychiatric problems associated with SUDs produce morbidity and mortality. These problems include the effects of intoxication, overdose, and withdrawal, and the consequences of chronic use. All organ systems are affected by SUDs. The following syndromes are among the major complications: gastritis, ulcers, pancreatitis, liver disease, cardiomyopathy, anemia, neurological complications, sexual dysfunction, fetal alcohol syndrome, and renal failure. Increased rates of oropharyngeal, esophageal, and hepatic cancer have been reported. Delirium tremens, intoxication, and other withdrawal syndromes can lead to death. The use of unsterile needles contributes to the spread of acquired immunodeficiency syndrome (AIDS), hepatitis, skin abscesses, endocarditis, mycotic aneurysms, septic arthritis, osteomyelitis, meningitis, and lung abscesses. And, not least, suicide remains a great complication of substance abuse.

AIDS and Intravenous Drugs

The intravenous use of opioids and cocaine has been a major risk factor in the spread of AIDS through needle sharing and disinhibition of risk-taking behavior. The latter includes promiscuous and "unsafe" sexual behavior. Either consciously or not, suicidal addicts may seek sexual partners and/or drug paraphernalia infected or contaminated with human immunodeficiency virus (HIV). Female addicts and female sexual partners of addicts who are HIV-positive have the added risk of spreading AIDS to their fetuses. Areas vary greatly in rates of infection and numbers of addicts at specific stages of the illness, with the urban poor and minorities being hardest hit by intravenous needle sharing. Continued intravenous use of cocaine in addicts maintained on methadone makes it harder to reduce HIV spread, even in relatively compliant methadone maintenance populations. Happily, by the end of the 1990s, with the introduction of the newest antiretroviral medications, there was evidence for a decline in the prevalence and incidence of HIV contracted by intravenous drug users.

Factors Contributing to Complications

Poor self-care, dietary problems (including poor nutrition and vitamin deficiencies), the use of unsterile needles, the admixture of unknown quantities of impure substances in the abused drug, and the psychosocial problems associated with addiction (e.g., increased personal risk of crime, suicidality, homicidality) contribute to medical and dental complications of drug abuse over and above the effects of the drug itself. The additional use of alcohol can further contribute to liver failure in intravenous drug users who have hepatitis and may lower resistance to infections and increase the risk of lung diseases (e.g., pneumonia, tuberculosis). Renal disease may be caused by antigen–antibody immune complexes resulting from infection and may be exacerbated by hypertension, which frequently accompanies substance abuse, especially alcohol and stimulant abuse. Cocaine use may contribute to hypertension, tachycardia, and arrhythmia and is a cause of sudden death. Patients with combinations of problems (e.g., alcohol withdrawal, diabetes, hypertension) who are given antidepressants may be at especially high risk for cardiac arrhythmias, vascular problems, and sudden death.

Chronic substance use can reduce sexual performance and desire in both sexes. Studies indicate that marijuana use as well as chronic alcohol use decrease serum testosterone in males.

Denial and Stigma

The patient with a substance use disorder may demonstrate denial, dissimulation, and memory problems related to organicity, as well as fear of stigmatization, making it difficult to obtain a clear history. Either because of refusal to cooperate or as a result of being socially isolated, the patient may not have family or friends who can be interviewed. Due to intoxication or overdose, the patient may be unable to answer coherently. Often, the patient who is seeking help has been coerced into seeing the doctor by family members, an employer, the court, or a family physician and has mixed feelings about cooperating. In addition to having a long-standing disrespect for authority figures that may have stemmed from being a child of an alcoholic, the patient may have had bad experiences with physicians who were not well informed about substance use problems. The patient needs reassurance that there is reason to be hopeful about the outcome of treatment, and an effort needs to be made to reduce blame and guilt. What the patient does not tell the doctor may be as important as what the patient does say; an alert clinician must watch for observable signs and symptoms as well as a mental status characterized by high denial, projection, and rationalization.

Facility Prejudices

Mentally ill patients who have SUDs are often inadequately managed in general psychiatric facilities and in freestanding alcohol and drug rehabilitation facilities that do not provide integrated treatment for patients with dual diagnoses. Minimal contact with the psychiatric consultant and primary treatment by alcoholism counselors, who may have insufficient psychiatric training, lead to underdiagnosis and insufficient treatment of additional psychiatric problems. For patients with psychosis, an abstinence-oriented program must be flexible, even when relapses occur. Many psychiatric halfway houses do not accept alcoholic patients, and halfway houses for substance abusers often do not accept patients on medications. Confrontational methods useful in therapeutic communities and self-help groups may be detrimental to those with more severe psychiatric illness. Full-service facilities with psychiatric treatment and rehabilitation are expensive; however, they represent a healthy integration of treatment approaches for mentally ill patients who abuse substances.

The Internet

The rise of the Internet has provided a tool through which those who abuse drugs can obtain information about drugs of abuse, including how to get them, how to hide them, how to grow plants, who to buy from and who not to buy from, how to cheat on drug tests, and where the interdiction agencies are concentrating their energies and attention. Most importantly, both illicit and controlled substances are sold over the Internet. This medium, which connects so many people, may do so for nefarious reasons! Nonetheless, information and connections gained over the Internet can be of great help to patients, families, and therapists (Table 2–1).

Key Points

- The societal effects of substances of abuse are vast.
- Rates of use of particular substances can vary greatly among specific demographic groups.
- Clinicians can refer to several up-to-date sources of information about substance use.

Table 2–1.   Helpful Internet sites

Addiction Resource Guide	www.addictionresourceguide.com
American Academy of Addiction Psychiatry	www.aaap.org
American Psychiatric Association	www.psych.org
Centers for Disease Control and Prevention *Morbidity and Mortality Weekly Report*	www.cdc.gov/mmwr
Centers for Disease Control and Prevention National Center for Health Statistics	www.cdc.gov/nchs
Centers for Disease Control and Prevention Office on Smoking and Health (OSH)	www.cdc.gov/tobacco
Council of State Governments Consensus Project	www.consensusproject.org
Monitoring the Future survey	www.monitoringthefuture.org
National Comorbidity Survey	www.hcp.med.harvard.edu/ncs
National Institute on Drug Abuse	www.drugabuse.gov
Office of National Drug Control Policy	www.whitehousedrugpolicy.gov
Substance Abuse and Mental Health Services Administration (includes National Survey on Drug Use and Health [NSDUH] and Drug Abuse Warning Network [DAWN])	www.samhsa.gov

References

Harwood H: Updating Estimates of the Economic Costs of Alcohol Abuse in the United States: Estimates, Update Methods, and Data. Report prepared by The Lewin Group for the National Institute on Alcohol Abuse and Alcoholism. Rockville, MD, National Institutes of Health, 2000 (Based on estimates, analyses, and data reported in Harwood H, Fountain D, Livermore G, et al: The Economic Costs of Alcohol and Drug Abuse in the United States 1992. Report prepared for the National Institute on Drug Abuse and the National Institute on Alcohol Abuse and Alcoholism, National Institutes of Health, Department of Health and Human Services. NIH Publ No 98-4327. Rockville, MD, National Institutes of Health, 1998)

Johnston LD, O'Malley PM, Bachman JG, et al: Monitoring the Future National Results on Adolescent Drug Use: Overview of Key Findings, 2007 (NIH Publ No 08-6418). Bethesda, MD, National Institute on Drug Abuse, 2008

Karch DL, Lubell KM, Friday KJ, et al: Surveillance for violent deaths—National Violent Death Reporting System, 16 states, 2005. MMWR Surveill Summ 57:1–45, 2008

Kessler RC, Crum RM, Warner LA, et al: Lifetime co-occurrence of DSM-III-R alcohol abuse and dependence with other psychiatric disorders in the National Comorbidity Survey. Arch Gen Psychiatry 54:313–321, 1997

Kessler RC, Chiu WT, Demler O, et al: Prevalence, severity, and comorbidity of 12-month DSM-IV disorders in the National Comorbidity Survey Replication. Arch Gen Psychiatry 62:617–627, 2005

National Highway Traffic Safety Administration: Traffic Safety Facts, 2006 Data: Alcohol-Impaired Driving (DOT HS 810 801). Washington, DC, National Highway Traffic Safety Administration, 2008

Regier DA, Farmer ME, Rae DS, et al: Co-morbidity of mental disorders with alcohol and other drug abuse: results from the Epidemiologic Catchment Area (ECA) Study. JAMA 264:2511–2518, 1990

Substance Abuse and Mental Health Services Administration, Center for Substance Abuse Treatment: Clinical Guidelines for the Use of Buprenorphine in the Treatment of Opioid Addiction. Treatment Improvement Protocol (TIP) Series 40; Publ No SMA 04-3939. Rockville, MD, U.S. Department of Health and Human Services, 2004a

Substance Abuse and Mental Health Services Administration: DAWN Report: Amphetamine and Methamphetamine Emergency Department Visits, 1995–2002. Rockville, MD, Office of Applied Studies, 2004b

Substance Abuse and Mental Health Services Administration: DAWN Report: Narcotic Analgesics, 2002 Update. Rockville, MD, Office of Applied Studies, 2004c

Substance Abuse and Mental Health Services Administration: Mortality Data From the Drug Abuse Warning Network, 2002 (DAWN Series D-25; DHHS Publ No SMA 04-3875). Rockville, MD, Office of Applied Studies, 2004d

Substance Abuse and Mental Health Services Administration: DAWN 2006: National Estimates of Drug-Related Emergency Department Visits (DAWN Series D-30; DHHS Publ No SMA 08-4339). Rockville, MD, Office of Applied Studies, 2008a

Substance Abuse and Mental Health Services Administration: Results From the 2007 National Survey on Drug Use and Health: National Findings (NSDUH Series H-34; DHHS Publ No SMA 08-4343). Rockville, MD, Office of Applied Studies, 2008b

Substance Abuse and Mental Health Services Administration: The NSDUH Report: Marijuana Use and Perceived Risk of Use Among Adolescents: 2002 to 2007. Rockville, MD, Office of Applied Studies, 2009a

Substance Abuse and Mental Health Services Administration: Results From the 2008 National Survey on Drug Use and Health: National Findings (NSDUH Series H-36; HHS Publ No SMA 09-4434). Rockville, MD, Office of Applied Studies, 2009b

3

Neurobiology of Addictive Disorders and the Disease Concept

In recent years, the assertion that substance abuse is simply a moral problem in which the choice to abuse a substance deserves more shame and punishment than empathy and treatment has been increasingly shown to be reductionistic and overly simplistic. An explosion of knowledge about the field has revealed that understanding addiction requires an understanding of a complex combination of factors. Conceptualizations of addiction as a disease may focus on homeostatic imbalance, discomfort, difference from the norm, discernible biological components, response to biological treatment, or lack of perfect health; definitions can be narrow or broad, culturally defined or universal, and can change over time. Currently, three (probably intertwined) perspectives on addiction are increasingly seen as central to an understanding of the condition: 1) addiction is the compulsion to use the substance, 2) addiction is a "brain disease," and 3) addiction is a chronic medical disorder.

That addiction is a "compulsion" means that the individual uses the substance at all costs, even in the face of severe negative consequences. As described later in this chapter, the evidence that there is a biological component to addiction is growing. The existence of biological markers provides a basis for genetic vulnerability to abuse particular substances. Furthermore, research is focusing on the long-term changes in synaptic architecture and alterations in neurotransmitter physiology that may form the basis of the position that the brain of the addicted patient is different as a result of excessive use—a difference that creates and maintains the compulsion to use (Leshner 1997). By no means should the perspective that addiction has a biological basis diminish the social, environmental, or personal aspects of addiction. However, biological evidence is important, at least in that it lends support to the disease model of addiction.

Another development in the conceptualization of addiction is in regard to the nature of the disease. Addictions have a chronic course, with multiple relapses. The individual abuser suffers from complications of use and also from social and economic problems as a result of abuse. More and more, practitioners involved in the treatment of addictions have noted parallels between substance use disorders (SUDs) and other chronic medical disorders such as diabetes mellitus, arthritis, or asthma—diseases that we can treat but perhaps never entirely cure, and in which relapses are to be expected, especially as they relate to choices patients make. In this view, the former cocaine abuser who relapses upon returning to the environment in which he or she previously used the drug is analogous to the child with asthma who develops an attack upon walking into a smoky room (O'Brien and McLellan 1996).

One implication of this view is that society ought to stop the moralizing that for generations has impeded recognition of, research in, and care for SUDs. Societal abandonment of the notion that dependence and abuse are the "fault" of the individual could lead to greater emphasis on treatment rather than punishment, reduction of overly harsh sentencing as dictated by statutes such as the "Rockefeller" drug laws in New York State, and use of drug courts and alternatives to sentencing that emphasize treatment for nonviolent drug crimes. On the other hand, such a perspective might be misconstrued as implying that abuse, dependence, or even relapse are acceptable and that abstinence is irrelevant—conclusions that could be used to support legalization of drug use. Most addiction and legal experts are against legalization, believing that it would lead to increased availability, increased craving, and increased prevalence and complications of addictions.

Ultimately, as with other chronic medical illnesses, the "cause" of addictive disorders should be seen as a combination of environment, genetics, and personal choice. With regard to personal choice, although addiction is an illness, there is an element of individual responsibility in seeking out and accepting help for recovery once a diagnosis is made. People are not robots, rats, or monkeys; even after becoming "hooked," addicted individuals can regain control over their lives by accepting an abstinence approach or (in the case of opioids) drug substitution (Committee on Addictions of the Group for the Advancement of Psychiatry 2002).

Nosology

Since the 1960s, American psychiatry has increasingly worked to improve the specificity of its classifications of mental disorders, in the hope that further refinement will lead to more precise characterizations of valid, distinct diseases. This thrust continues in the DSM-IV era (American Psychiatric Association 1994). Both DSM-IV and its Text Revision, DSM-IV-TR (American Psychiatric Association 2000), provide specifiers to be used to differentiate between alcohol dependence with a physiological component (i.e., tolerance or withdrawal) and alcohol dependence without such a component. A study of 3,395 alcohol-dependent individuals suggested that physical dependence, especially when marked by symptoms of withdrawal, predicts a more severe course of alcoholism (Schuckit et al. 1998). Thus, researchers continue the attempt to define addiction and to delineate its various types.

Neurobiology of the Addictions: Clinical Implications of Research Findings

Major developments at the end of the 1990s included the elucidation of the neural circuits by which addiction was mediated; an important brain circuit activated by opioids as well as other abused drugs is the mesolimbic system. An area of the brain known as the ventral tegmental area signals another part of the brain, the nucleus accumbens, via the inhibitory neurotransmitter dopamine.

A behavior that results in the release of dopamine into the nucleus accumbens will be reinforced, hence this circuitry is often referred to as the "reward circuitry." Other areas of the brain create lasting memories that associate the reinforcing feelings with the circumstances and environment in which they occur, and these memories can be triggers for relapse later on during recovery. This same brain pathway is activated by other abused drugs, but often via different mechanisms. For example, opioids and cannabinoids can inhibit activity in nucleus accumbens directly. Stimulants such as cocaine and amphetamine act indirectly by binding to various dopamine transporters. In the case of cocaine, this inhibits the reuptake of dopamine into the ventral tegmental area neurons, whereas with amphetamine, dopamine is actively pumped out of the ventral tegmental area into the nucleus accumbens. As drug use continues over time, the neurons become affected in such a way that more and more of the drug is needed to release the same amount of dopamine. This results in the clinical phenomenon known as tolerance.

Genetics: Familial Studies and High-Risk Populations

Beyond circuitry, the genetic studies since the late 1990s have elucidated ever more information. Family studies have demonstrated that there is familial transmission of a propensity not just to a particular substance of abuse, but probably to addiction in general. People with alcohol dependence are not only more likely to have relatives in their families who are also dependent on alcohol, but they are more likely to have relatives with dependence on other substances such as cocaine, heroin, and tobacco. The risk of alcohol dependence in relatives of proband alcohol-dependent patients compared with control subjects is about twofold (Nurnberger et al. 2004). Although it could be argued that familial patterns of addiction could be related to a variety of social and environmental variables, twin studies have demonstrated that considerable variability in risk for developing addiction is due to genetics. Yet, among unaffected monozygotic twins reared in a nonabusing household, the risk of alcohol misuse was no greater among control subjects, suggesting that environment matters (Jacob et al. 2003). There are clear genetic factors in the ability to maintain abstinence.

There is evidence that various phenomena associated with alcohol use, particularly flushing and blackouts, also have a genetic component. The flushing response occurs in Asian populations and is the result of a single-point mutation and may protect that group from excessive alcohol intake. In some cultures, the flushing response reduces drinking; in others, such as Korean populations, it does not. Blackouts, or anterograde amnesia following a period of heavy drinking, occur in a large percentage of people who do not necessarily have alcohol dependence. Blackouts appear to be the result of γ-aminobutyric acid (GABA)–mediated inhibition of neural activity, as well as antagonism at the N-methyl-D-aspartate (NMDA)–mediated glutamate receptors. Twin studies have demonstrated that there is a significant genetic component to the risk of experiencing blackouts in one's lifetime (Nelson et al. 2004).

That alcoholism occurs in families was established 70 years ago by Jellinek and Jolliffe (1940). In alcohol dependence, genetic influences are greater in early-onset than in late-onset dependence (Liu et al. 2004). Although genetic influences in alcoholism and other drug abuse patterns in both men and women have become fairly well established through twin, adoption, and split-sibling studies, neither the mode of transmission nor the exact nature of what is being transmitted is clear. In regard to alcohol dependence, some studies have suggested that tolerance to alcohol is the transmitted trait. In establishing the genetic bases of cocaine and cannabis abuse, other studies have proposed that there is a general vulnerability to a particular substance that is transmitted, such that a person with that vulnerability might become addicted after only one exposure (Nurnberger et al. 2004). Additional studies have focused on abnormalities in dopamine receptor subtypes in the nucleus accumbens, the ventral striatum, NMDA glutamate receptors, alcohol dehydrogenase (ADH2*2 allele as protective), neuropeptide Y (Pro7 allele), and others (Galanter and Kleber 2008).

Further lines of research in the genetics of the addictions will address variability among patients; pharmacogenetics and gender differences in genetic transmission are two important topics. A greater understanding of genetics could lead to better efforts at prevention, and understanding of the pathogenesis of addiction could lead to new treatments. These findings are not limited to alcohol. The literature includes data about the moderate genetic impact on most cannabis use, which is seen as stronger at more severe levels of use (Hopfer et al. 2003). And, there is an increased interest in genetic influences on nicotine dependence—but the impact on initiation and regular use are higher than they are for the diagnosis of nicotine dependence (Maes et al. 2004).

Biological Markers

Biological markers are associated, if not causal, findings that may help us to identify high-risk individuals before the onset of abuse, identify dependence when it does exist, and follow the course of the disease (see Chapter 4, "Evaluation and Assessment"). In addition, the drug of abuse becomes more salient than other rewards, such as money, and this change in behavior can be correlated with changes in brain activation on functional magnetic resonance imaging (fMRI). In particular, the prefrontal-orbitofrontal-cortical circuit has been shown to be involved in this change in salience seen in addicted patients (Goldstein et al. 2007).

Identifying children at high risk for alcoholism or substance abuse has been one major research thrust. Schuckit (1987) and his group have studied multiple markers in biological sons of alcoholics (Table 3–1). Findings have included evidence of decreased subjective feelings of intoxication in not-yet-alcoholic children of alcoholics and of less impairment of motor performance (including less body sway or static ataxia) with alcohol challenge in comparison with control subjects, as well as less change in cortisol and prolactin levels. Clinicians working with adolescent or young adult populations should focus closely on the young patient's initial experiences with alcohol. Does the adolescent drink much more than peers without showing signs or symptoms of intoxication? What is the best advice for a young person who experiences few adverse effects from drinking but who has a strong family history of dependence? An early choice of abstinence may be the safest form of prevention for such an individual. Often, these teenagers will describe their first encounter with alcohol as a revelation, an "ah ha" experience in which alcohol is discovered as an ideal way to handle anxiety, decrease stress, and express emotions.

Electroencephalographic Markers

A finding among abstinent alcoholics and sons of alcoholics is an alteration of normal auditory brainstem potentials. The P300 event-related potential (the voltage of the third positive electroencephalography [EEG] wave in response to this stimulus) is of low amplitude in alcoholics and abstinent young sons of alcoholic men. The P300 component may be related to motivational properties of stimuli and may be involved in the process of memory. The association with alcoholism is well replicated, but the finding is not limited to

Table 3–1. Possible markers of alcoholism in biological sons of alcoholics

Decreased subjective feelings of intoxication

Less impairment of motor performance

Less body sway

Less static ataxia

Less change in cortisol and prolactin findings

Low P300 amplitude (electroencephalogram)

Increased alpha-wave activity

alcoholics or their children. Thus, although specificity of this possible marker is not high enough for predictive value, this is a promising area of research. Increased alpha-wave activity with alcohol exposure in biological sons of alcoholics versus control subjects has also been reported (see Table 3–1). Abnormal P300 component findings might be more valid for visual stimuli than for auditory stimuli (Polich and Bloom 1999). These findings may reflect brainstem demyelination. A heritable reduction in P300 occurs in women with alcoholism, independent of depression (Suresh et al. 2003).

Alcohol Metabolism

Alcohol dehydrogenase and aldehyde dehydrogenase are the two hepatic enzymes involved in metabolism of ethanol. Current research is attempting to learn how the five genes that make up alcohol dehydrogenase (which are transmitted on the long arm of chromosome 4) could be correlated with the threefold variability known to exist in ethanol metabolism among humans.

Ethanol is an NMDA receptor antagonist; therefore, it is reasonable to suggest that the glutamatergic system is likely to be involved in alcohol abuse and dependence. There is growing evidence to suggest that this is, in fact, the case. Compared with control subjects, patients who have a family history of alcoholism show variations in their emotional response to ketamine, a drug that is also an NMDA receptor antagonist. Numerous animal studies and imaging studies support the idea that this circuit is necessary for drug-seeking behavior to occur (Daglish et al. 2001), and this raises new possibilities about potential targets for pharmacological treatment of addiction.

Even after the onset of abstinence, patients with a history of alcohol dependence show differences in their brain functioning compared with healthy control subjects. Chronic alcohol use leads to downregulation of central D_2 receptors. Delayed recovery of D_2 receptor sensitivity following detoxification from alcohol is associated with a greater risk of relapse. Functional imaging studies have demonstrated that this delayed recovery of receptors leads to decreased D_2 receptor availability in the ventral striatum and nucleus accumbens (Heinz et al. 2004). When exposed to a trigger to drink, such as a photograph of someone ingesting alcohol, a patient with a history of alcoholism will have decreased stimulation in these areas of the brain associated with reward, and will therefore have craving for alcohol.

Neurochemical Markers

There has been controversy over whether there is low activity of platelet monoamine oxidase B (MAO-B) in alcohol-dependent individuals. Low platelet MAO-B activity has been observed; it may be more pronounced in Type II alcoholism than in Type I. The low activity has been noted to persist despite abstinence; nonetheless, it may be more a marker of state than of trait (Coccini et al. 2002). Adenylate cyclase in platelets and lymphocytes has also been studied and is usually shown to be reduced in alcoholics, although the significance of this finding is unknown.

Neuropsychological Performance

Prospective longitudinal studies of sons of alcoholics have shown some evidence of poor neuropsychological performance in areas such as categorizing ability, organization, planning, abstracting, and problem-solving ability. Tarter and Edwards (1988) suggested that minimal brain dysfunction or conduct disorder may predispose an individual to alcoholism and may be an expression of an underlying inherited temperament. Risk-taking, sensation-seeking individuals are thought to be at particularly high risk. Cocaine intoxication involves altered perceptions, which can include those regarding the value of money (Goldstein et al. 2007).

The insula, a part of the brain that is associated with conscious urges, is another part of the brain that has been suggested to be involved with addiction, at least with regard to nicotine. This hypothesis developed after investigators found that cigarette smokers who suffered brain injuries that involved the insula were more likely to quit smoking than smokers who had suffered brain injuries that did not involve the insula (Naqvi et al. 2007). These smokers found it easy to quit immediately and did not suffer from craving or relapse.

Cellular Pathophysiology of Addiction

Over the past few decades, advances in cellular and molecular biology have been astonishing, and this is no less the case in psychiatry and the addictions. There is increasing evidence that craving of and addiction to virtually all substances of abuse (even cannabinoids [Diana et al. 1998]) are related to the dopaminergic systems in the brain—especially the mesolimbic reward system and the areas to which it projects: the limbic system and the orbitofrontal cortex (Leshner and Koob 1999). This may be due not only to homeostatic adaptations of neurons but also to neural plasticity and synaptic rearrangement that result from activation of particular signal transduction pathways between stimulus and gene expression.

The idea is that addiction is not just a degenerative disease or a lesion but also a learned process in which long-term memory occurs (inappropriately) at the molecular level. Such a view reduces the serious nature of relapse (O'Brien and McLellan 1996). It will be necessary in the future to study mechanisms of molecular memory and their relation to decreasing addiction.

As noted earlier, there is evidence that the compulsion to use particular substances is the result of craving that comes from an environmental cue. Compulsion is at least partly seated in the mesolimbic system, although various avenues of investigation are focused on delineating the effects of genetic variants—such as those of cannabinoid receptor type 1 (CB_1)—on risk of use (Hutchison et al. 2008). It is recognized that the CB_1 receptor, a G protein–coupled receptor, is located in the same anatomic sites as those recognized to be involved in addiction. Genetic variation is seen as an avenue to understanding, as alterations in gene expression have resulted in alterations in substance use. Further study has focused on the interaction of CB_1 with nicotine dependence (Chen et al. 2008). Animals with the gene for CB_1 (or *CNR1*) knocked out have altered responses to nicotine, ethanol, cocaine, amphetamine, and other psychostimulants. At the same time, there is interest in the variants of the nicotinic acetylcholine receptors as mediators of compulsive use (Thorgeirsson and Stefansson 2008).

Key Points

- Addictive disorders are chronic medical conditions that involve genetic, environmental, and personal choices as influences.
- Addiction utilizes the neural reward circuitry that evolved in humans to encourage behavior that is beneficial, such as eating or mating.
- The reward circuitry involves dopamine release in the nucleus accumbens, which signals the brain that the stimulus is "salient."
- Glutamatergic projections from the nucleus accumbens to the prefrontal cortex seem to be the final common pathway for the neural circuitry that mediates drug-seeking behavior.

References

American Psychiatric Association: Diagnostic and Statistical Manual of Mental Disorders, 4th Edition. Washington, DC, American Psychiatric Association, 1994

American Psychiatric Association: Diagnostic and Statistical Manual of Mental Disorders, 4th Edition, Text Revision. Washington, DC, American Psychiatric Association, 2000

Chen X, Williamson VS, An SS, et al: Cannabinoid receptor 1 gene association with nicotine dependence. Arch Gen Psychiatry 65:816–824, 2008

Coccini T, Castoldi AF, Gandini C, et al: Platelet monoamine oxidase B activity as a state marker for alcoholism: trend over time during withdrawal and influence of smoking and gender. Alcohol Alcohol 37:566–572, 2002

Committee on Addictions of the Group for the Advancement of Psychiatry: Responsibility and choice in addiction. Psychiatr Serv 53:707–713, 2002

Daglish MR, Weinstein A, Malizia AL, et al: Changes in regional cerebral blood flow elicited by craving memories in abstinent opiate-dependent subjects. Am J Psychiatry 158:1680–1686, 2001

Diana M, Melis M, Muntoni AL, et al: Meso-limbic dopaminergic decline after cannabinoid withdrawal. Proc Natl Acad Sci U S A 95:10269–10273, 1998

Galanter M, Kleber HD (eds): The American Psychiatric Publishing Textbook of Substance Abuse Treatment, 4th Edition. Washington, DC, American Psychiatric Publishing, 2008

Goldstein RZ, Alia-Klein N, Tomasi D, et al: Is decreased prefrontal cortical sensitivity to monetary reward associated with impaired motivation and self-control in cocaine addiction? Am J Psychiatry 164:43–51, 2007

Heinz A, Siessmeier T, Wrase J, et al: Correlation between dopamine D(2) receptors in the ventral striatum and central processing of alcohol cues and craving. Am J Psychiatry 161:1783–1789, 2004

Hopfer CJ, Stallings MC, Hewitt JK, et al: Family transmission of marijuana use, abuse, and dependence. J Am Acad Child Adolesc Psychiatry 42:834–841, 2003

Hutchison KE, Haughey H, Niculescu M, et al: The incentive salience of alcohol: translating the effects of genetic variant in CNR1. Arch Gen Psychiatry 65:841–850, 2008

Jacob T, Waterman B, Heath A, et al: Genetic and environmental effects on offspring alcoholism: new insights using an offspring of twins design. Arch Gen Psychiatry 60:1265–1272, 2003

Jellinek EM, Jolliffe N: Effect of alcohol on the individual: review of the literature of 1939. Q J Stud Alcohol 1:110–181, 1940

Leshner AI: Addiction is a brain disease and it matters. Science 278:45–47, 1997

Leshner AI, Koob GF: Drugs of abuse and the brain. Proc Assoc Am Physicians 111:99–108, 1999

Liu IC, Blacker DL, Zu R, et al: Genetic and environmental contributions to the development of alcohol dependence in male twins. Arch Gen Psychiatry 61:897–903, 2004

Maes HH, Sullivan PF, Bulik CM, et al: A twin study of genetic and environmental influences on tobacco initiation, regular tobacco use, and nicotine dependence. Psychol Med 34:1251–1261, 2004

Naqvi NH, Rudrauf D, Damasio H, et al: Damage to the insula disrupts addiction to cigarette smoking. Science 315:531–534, 2007

Nelson EC, Heath AC, Bucholz KK, et al: Genetic epidemiology of alcohol induced blackouts. Arch Gen Psychiatry 61:257–263, 2004

Nurnberger JI Jr, Wiegland R, Buholz K, et al: A family study of alcohol dependence: coaggregation of multiple disorders in relatives of alcohol dependent probands. Arch Gen Psychiatry 61:1246–1256, 2004

O'Brien CP, McLellan AT: Myths about the treatment of addiction. Lancet 347:237–240, 1996

Polich J, Bloom FE: P300, alcoholism heritablility, and stimulus modality. Alcohol 17:149–156, 1999

Schuckit MA: Biological vulnerability to alcoholism. J Consult Clin Psychol 55:301–309, 1987

Schuckit MA, Smith TL, Daeppen JB, et al: Clinical relevance of the distinction between alcohol dependence with and without a physiological component. Am J Psychiatry 155:733–740, 1998

Suresh S, Porjesz B, Chorlian DB, et al: Auditory P3 in female alcoholics. Alcohol Clin Exp Res 27:1064–1074, 2003

Tarter RE, Edwards K: Psychological factors associated with the risk for alcoholism. Alcohol Clin Exp Res 12:471–480, 1988

Thorgeirsson TE, Stefansson K: Genetics of smoking behavior and its consequences: the role of nicotinic acetylcholine receptors. Biol Psychiatry 64:919–921, 2008

4

Evaluation and Assessment

A Moving Target

Assessment is a continuous process that occurs in every interaction with a substance-using patient. The various facets of a patient's status may be changing at all times; the clinician should follow, among other aspects of status, motivation/readiness for change, withdrawal status, and stability of co-occurring psychiatric disorders. Assessment, like any part of medicine, involves some combination of history, examination, and other studies, ranging from general to specific instruments, imaging, or blood/chemistry. The form and content of assessment vary according to setting (e.g., emergency department, outpatient psychiatric care, methadone maintenance program, intensive care unit) and phase of recovery (e.g., detoxification, case identification, remission). Of course, the clinician should consider a patient's age, culture, and ethnicity, as well as psychiatric and medical status. Diagnosis (as described in Chapter 5, "Definition, Presentation, and Diagnosis") is but one piece of the puzzle—a good assessment will evaluate and describe the relevant problem areas and individual texture in each patient's presentation.

Admission Workup

In the general hospital setting, detailed alcohol and other substance use histories should be taken from every patient at admission. Information should be gathered in a straightforward manner in concert with the rest of the medical history. When substance use problems do exist, the patient's answers may be vague, evasive, or aggressively defensive. In early abuse patterns, some patients may be surprised by the connection between their substance use and their current medical problems. Health professionals should be familiar with the components of a basic alcohol and other substance use history (Table 4–1). Due to the potential for denial and resistance, organicity, and psychiatric symptoms, a consultation with an addiction specialist may be helpful in making a diagnosis. Third-party sources such as family or friends may be needed to obtain crucial information. For example, additional corroboration was necessary for assessment of prior alcohol abuse in a man who had been admitted for routine surgery and denied alcohol abuse on admission but appeared to be in early stages of delirium tremens 2 days later. The psychoactive substance abuse history should be a systematic review of all the major drug classes. Often, patients will not consider a particular substance to be "a drug." For example, a 30-year-old woman who had been smoking marijuana every day since college did not consider marijuana to be a drug, but rather an herbal remedy. The query "Do you abuse drugs?" seemed to her pejorative. She did not offer the desired information due to a lack of knowledge and her particular view of the stigma of drug abuse. Another example is Rastafarians, who view use of marijuana as part of their religious beliefs.

Specific Substance Use History-Taking

Experience with drug classes such as alcohol, opioids, cocaine, or other stimulants, tranquilizers, hallucinogens, marijuana, inhalants, and over-the-counter medications should be systematically ascertained. Use and possible abuse of prescription medications should be explored. Patient history should include the type of liquor or specific drug used; amount, pattern, or frequency of use; and time of last use. Recent historical information may be very important in distinguishing various organic mental states. In addition, the patient's route of administration (oral, intravenous, or pulmonary inhalation) may

Table 4–1. Components of a basic alcohol and other substance use history

Chief complaint

Current medical signs and symptoms

Substance abuse review of systems for all substances of abuse

Dates of first use, regular use, longest period of sobriety and overall life condition during sobriety, pattern, amount, frequency, time of last use, route of administration, circumstances of use, reactions to use

Medical history, medications, HIV and TB status

History of past substance abuse treatment, response to treatment, history of complications secondary to substances

Psychiatric history

Family history of psychiatric disease and substance use

Legal history

Object relations history

Personal and social history

Review of collected data (chart, family, primary care physician)

Note. HIV = human immunodeficiency virus; TB = tuberculosis.

have important health consequences. For example, human immunodeficiency virus (HIV) screening should be done on the vast majority of intravenous drug addicts who present for admission in the general hospital setting. If alcohol abuse is suspected, symptoms of physical dependence must be actively pursued. Missing such information can be life-threatening.

A history of early-morning tremors or shakes, a subjective need for a drink to calm the nerves, elevated pulse and blood pressure, or a known history of alcohol-related seizures or delirium tremens should signal the need for pharmacological detoxification. Polysubstance abuse may mask underlying physical dependence on one prominent psychoactive substance (e.g., opioids in "speedballing" [mixing cocaine and heroin] or "hits" [combined use of heroin and cocaine]; alcohol dependence secondary to cocaine addiction). The patient should be asked about any past hospitalizations for motor vehicle accidents, accidental injuries, or substance-related violence, in addition to any history of treatment for alcohol or other substance abuse problems. Any intoxicated patient should be seen as potentially violent to self or others. Addressing nutritional and metabolic status is of particular importance for persons who have been misusing substances over time; Wernicke-Korsakoff syndrome is but one example of the effects of malnutrition from a substance use disorder.

Diagnostic Instruments

Attempts to identify definitive psychological features of individuals who abuse alcohol and substances have generally failed. Early psychodynamic theorists described addictive behavior as related to oral-regressive defense mechanisms. More recently, theorists have discussed ego disturbances, difficulty with affect regulation, and defective self-care mechanisms. Pathological dependency, feelings of inadequacy, and counterdependency feelings of bravado have been described in these patients. Furthermore, a "temperament" of risk taking, sensation seeking, and compulsivity has also been correlated with high levels of substance abuse.

Cognitive theorists have posited that psychoactive substance abuse provides tension and stress reduction, positive expectancy of mood elevation, and increased perception of self-adequacy. While comorbidity with other Axis I disorders is frequent, no one alcohol or substance abuse personality has proved to be etiological, although substance abuse is overrepresented in those with personality disorders, particularly in persons with antisocial and borderline personality disorders.

Instruments Used in Research

The need for better standardized diagnostic research instruments in psychiatry has produced structured interviews that have been helpful in identifying alcoholism in large epidemiological studies. These instruments are also used to identify a variety of psychiatric diagnoses, both substance use disorders and others. The Schedule for Affective Disorders and Schizophrenia (SADS), based on the Research Diagnostic Criteria, is a forerunner to the Diagnostic Interview Schedule (DIS). The DIS, based on DSM-IV (American Psychiatric Association 1994) criteria, is an instrument designed to be administered by trained lay interviewers. The Structured Clinical Interview for DSM-IV (SCID) is a more recent structured interview (also based on DSM-IV criteria) that can also be used to make DSM-IV personality disorder diagnoses. These instruments have proved to be fairly reliable in establishing DSM-IV and Research Diagnostic Criteria psychoactive substance abuse diagnoses. However, problems may exist in assessing other psychiatric diagnoses with these instruments in the psychoactive substance abuse population. In particular, the anxiety, antisocial, and depression sections may be less useful for diagnoses in this population.

There are several instruments designed for research purposes that finely measure attributes of alcohol abuse. The Alcohol Use Inventory is a 17-item, self-administered questionnaire that assesses 1) the perceived benefits of alcohol, 2) the problems concomitant with alcohol use, 3) the disruptive consequences of drinking, and 4) the patient's concern about the use of alcohol and the extent to which the patient acknowledges having a drinking problem. The Alcohol Dependence Scale is a 10-question instrument assessing physical dependence.

Dimensional Scales

Dimensional personality profile scales such as the Minnesota Multiphasic Personality Inventory (MMPI) and the Symptom Checklist (SCL)–90 have been useful in substance abuse populations. In the hands of a skilled interpreter, common findings of elevated scores on hysteria, paranoia, antisocial, and depression subscales can augment initial clinical impressions. A markedly elevated schizophrenia scale score or evidence of gender identity confusion may occasionally be expected. Profiles may indicate that the patient is dissimulating to fake good or bad scores. Although its usefulness is limited to augmentation of a good clinical diagnostic interview, the MMPI may be most helpful for charting improvement over time. Due to the time-limited physiological effects of alcohol, patients' symptoms frequently begin to clear after 3 or 4 weeks of abstinence, and this is reflected in the test. Personality subscales may improve as the acquired substance abuse–related personality attributes begin to clear. Conversely, serious psychiatric problems may also be unmasked following drug removal. Frequently, damage to personality structure improves, but recovery may not be total. The MacAndrew Alcoholism Scale, a 49-question true/false subscale of the MMPI, has been widely used in the assessment of alcoholic patients. Although this scale has shown promise (correctly identifying 82% of those with alcoholism; MacAndrew 1965), more recent studies have highlighted some of its limitations in the general medical population.

Screening Instruments

There are several instruments designed to measure various aspects of alcohol and other substance abuse. Most of these instruments are not based on research criteria but have been found to be clinically useful in identifying psychoactive substance abuse. Two widely used alcoholism screening tests are the Michigan Alcoholism Screening Test (MAST; Selzer 1971) (Table 4–2) and the CAGE Questionnaire (Ewing 1984) (Table 4–3). These tests have the advantage of being self-administered, brief screens that can point the way for further study. The MAST is a 25-question form. The Short MAST (SMAST) is a 13-item scale that correlates 0.90 with the MAST. The MAST has a test–retest reliability in excess of 0.85. The sensitivities of the MAST and the SMAST are approximately 0.90 and 0.70, respectively. The proportion of nonalcoholics correctly identified as such averages 0.74 for the MAST. These tests screen for the major psychological, social, and physiological consequences of alcoholism.

The "One-Question Screen" developed by the National Institute on Alcohol Abuse and Alcoholism (2007) may be useful for the busy clinician who is trying to evaluate many syndromes besides substance use. In this screen, patients are asked a single question: "How many times in the past year have you had 5 or more drinks [or, for women, 4 or more drinks] in the same day?" The screen is considered positive for any answer greater than 0, and the clinician is prompted to explore further.

Addiction Severity Index

The Addiction Severity Index (developed by McLellan et al. 1992) has proved to be a useful instrument in the substance abuse population, particularly in treatment outcome research (Rikoon et al. 2006). It establishes a scale and scoring system for the severity of need for treatment in seven major areas: medical status, employment and support, drug use, alcohol use, legal status, family or social status, and psychiatric status. This dimensional approach is most helpful in identifying treatment needs when attempting to match the patient with a specific tailored treatment. The instrument can be administered by any trained person and takes approximately 50–60 minutes to administer. In addition, there is an Addiction Severity Index geared toward teenagers (Kaminer et al. 1991).

Substance-Specific Assessment Instruments

Several groups have developed assessment tools targeted toward a particular substance of abuse. The following list suggests a few noteworthy instruments for assessment of substance use:

- The Alcohol Use Disorders Identification Test (AUDIT; Babor et al. 2001) is a written self-report instrument that screens for harmful or hazardous alcohol use (Table 4–4); it has high levels of validity and reliability (Reinert and Allen 2002).
- TWEAK, named for the five items for which it screens (Tolerance, Worried, Eye-opener, Amnesia, K[C]ut down), was originally developed to identify high-risk drinking during pregnancy; it has been validated in both male and female populations (Dawson et al. 2001).
- T-ACE (Tolerance, Annoyed, Cut down, Eye opener), a 4-item screening questionnaire based on the CAGE assessment tool, was developed to identify pregnant women who may be drinking in quantities that are dangerous to the fetus (Russell 1994).
- The Fagerström Test for Nicotine Dependence, a 6-item test, measures nicotine dependence (Sledjeski et al. 2007).

Substance-Specific Withdrawal Instruments

As discussed in Chapter 13 ("Treatment Approaches"), numerous instruments have been developed to assist in assessment and monitoring of individuals who are experiencing withdrawal, and clinicians may find these useful in calibrating interventions. They include the following:

- *Alcohol:* Clinical Institute Withdrawal Assessment for Alcohol—Revised (CIWA-Ar; Sullivan et al. 1989)
- *Opioids:* Clinical Institute Narcotic Assessment (CINA) scale (Fudala et al. 1991) and Clinical Opiate Withdrawal Scale (COWS; Wesson and Ling 2003)
- *Cocaine:* Cocaine Selective Severity Assessment (CSSA; Kampman et al. 1998)

Table 4–2. Michigan Alcoholism Screening Test (MAST)

Points	Question	Yes	No
	0. Do you enjoy a drink now and then?		
(2)	1. Do you feel you are a normal drinker? (By normal we mean you drink less than or as much as most other people).		
(2)	2. Have you ever awakened the morning after some drinking the night before and found that you could not remember a part of the evening?		
(1)	3. Does your wife, husband, parent, or other near relative ever worry or complain about your drinking?		
(2)	4. Can you stop drinking without a struggle after one or two drinks?		
(1)	5. Do you ever feel guilty about your drinking?		
(2)	6. Do friends or relatives think you are a normal drinker?		
(0)	7. Do you ever try to limit your drinking to certain times of the day or to certain places?		
(2)	8. Have you ever attended a meeting of Alcoholics Anonymous?		
(1)	9. Have you gotten into physical fights when drinking?		
(2)	10. Has your drinking ever created problems between you and your wife, husband, a parent, or other relative?		
(2)	11. Has your wife or husband (or other family members) ever gone to anyone for help about your drinking?		
(2)	12. Have you ever lost friends because of your drinking?		
(2)	13. Have you ever gotten into trouble at work or school because of drinking?		
(2)	14. Have you ever lost a job because of drinking?		
(2)	15. Have you ever neglected your obligations, your family, or your work for 2 or more days in a row because you were drinking?		
(1)	16. Do you drink before noon fairly often?		

Table 4–2. Michigan Alcoholism Screening Test (MAST) *(continued)*

Points	Question	Yes	No
(2)	17. Have you ever been told you have liver trouble? Cirrhosis?	—	—
(2)	*18. After heavy drinking, have you ever had delirium tremens (DTs), severe shaking, or heard voices or seen things that really were not there?	—	—
(5)	19. Have you ever gone to anyone for help about your drinking?	—	—
(5)	20. Have you ever been in a hospital because of drinking?	—	—
(2)	21. Have you ever been a patient in a psychiatric hospital or on a psychiatric ward of a general hospital where drinking was part of the problem that resulted in hospitalization?	—	—
(2)	22. Have you ever been seen at a psychiatric or mental health clinic or gone to any doctor, social worker, or clergyman for help with any emotional problem where drinking was part of the problem?	—	—
(2)	**23. Have you ever been arrested for drunk driving, driving while intoxicated, or driving under the influence of alcoholic beverages? (If YES, How many times?___)	—	—
(2)	**24. Have you ever been arrested or taken into custody—even for a few hours—because of other drunk behavior? (If YES, How many times? ___)	—	—

*Five points for DTs; **Two points for each arrest.

Scoring system: In general, 5 points or more would place the subject in an "alcoholic" category, 4 points would suggest alcoholism, and 3 points or less would indicate the subject is not alcoholic.

Programs using the above scoring system find it very sensitive at the 5-point level and it tends to find more people alcoholics than anticipated. However, it is a screening test and should be sensitive at its lower levels.

Source. Reprinted with permission from Selzer ML: "The Michigan Alcoholism Screening Test: The Quest for a New Diagnostic Instrument." *American Journal of Psychiatry* 127:1653–1658, 1971. Copyright 1971, American Psychiatric Association.

Table 4–3.   CAGE Questionnaire

Scores: 2–3: High index of suspicion; 4: pathognomonic

Have you ever:

C   Thought you should CUT back on your drinking?

A   Felt ANNOYED by people criticizing your drinking?

G   Felt GUILTY or bad about your drinking

E   Had a morning EYE OPENER to relieve hangover or nerves?

Source.   Reproduced with permission from Ewing JA: "Detecting Alcoholism: The CAGE Questionnaire." *Journal of the American Medical Association* 252:1905–1907, 1984. Copyright 1984, American Medical Association.

Laboratory Evaluations

Laboratory evaluations are only one part of a full evaluation, but in the care of addicted patients they carry a great deal of weight. Laboratory evaluations may be done for a variety of purposes, including the following:

- to supplement information obtained in drug histories, which is often of poor quality
- because laboratory results are likely to correlate with clinical state
- to clarify differential diagnosis
- as part of follow-up
- as part of assessment
- for forensic needs
- to test athletes
- to enforce public safety (for high-responsibility jobs)
- to detect relapse
- to deter drug use (routine testing)
- to encourage sobriety
- to screen job applicants
- to identify recent use

Urine and Blood Screens

In the absence of a clear history of substance use disorder, several physical signs or laboratory test results may suggest the presence of a primary substance abuse disorder. General findings that should heighten suspicion of drug abuse in unknown cases include the following: vital sign changes; abnormal pupil size or conjunctival injection; tremor; diaphoresis; agitation, irritability, or unpredictable behavior; needle marks or scars; and evidence of unexplained trauma. Inadequate management of pain with unusual analgesic dosages and unexpected elevated blood levels of commonly abused substances (e.g., alcohol) without obvious intoxication may also signal drug or alcohol tolerance and addiction. Most commonly abused drugs are included in the typical drug screen, but if clinical presentation suggests a particular drug, that substance may need to be screened for specifically.

The importance of urine and blood level tests as a means of screening for and providing collateral evidence for substance abuse problems cannot be overstressed. The sensitivity and accuracy of blood and urine screening has improved with the addition of gas chromatography to more routine screening techniques. A general toxicology screen includes a blood alcohol level test.

Blood alcohol level can be helpful in assessing the likelihood of alcohol withdrawal. The presence of withdrawal signs at higher blood alcohol levels is suggestive of a severe impending withdrawal state. It should be recalled that alcohol intoxication is not simply based on blood alcohol level; tolerant individuals may have a high blood alcohol level in the absence of clinically significant intoxication.

Selection of Toxicological Tests and Pharmacokinetics

There are five points to consider when choosing a test:

1. Which substance(s) to sample
2. Half-life of the suspected substance(s)
3. Significance of biotransformation of the suspected substance(s)
4. Sensitivity and specificity of the test
5. Cost

Knowledge of the half-life of various drug doses will be helpful in making sense of test results. For example, 4 ounces of orally administered ethyl alcohol will have a half-life of 1–2 hours. A blood alcohol level of 200 mg/dL would indicate recent heavy intake and most likely current intoxication. A negative paper chromatography drug screen for cocaine in a man admitted for

Table 4–4.   Alcohol Use Disorders Identification Test (AUDIT)

Questions	0	1	2	3	4
1. How often do you have a drink containing alcohol?	Never	Monthly	2–4 times a month	2–3 times a week	4 or more times a week
2. How many drinks containing alcohol do you have on a typical day when you are drinking?	1 or 2	3 or 4	5 or 6	7 to 9	10 or more
3. How often do you have 5 or more drinks on one occasion?	Never	Less than monthly	Monthly	Weekly	Daily or almost daily
4. How often during the last year have you found that you were not able to stop drinking once you had started?	Never	Less than monthly	Monthly	Weekly	Daily or almost daily
5. How often during the last year have you failed to do what was normally expected of you because of drinking?	Never	Less than monthly	Monthly	Weekly	Daily or almost daily
6. How often during the last year have you needed a first drink in the morning to get yourself going after a heavy drinking session?	Never	Less than monthly	Monthly	Weekly	Daily or almost daily
7. How often during the last year have you had a feeling of guilt or remorse after drinking?	Never	Less than monthly	Monthly	Weekly	Daily or almost daily
8. How often during the last year have you been unable to remember what happened the night before because of drinking?	Never	Less than monthly	Monthly	Weekly	Daily or almost daily
9. Have you or someone else been injured because of your drinking?	No		Yes, but not in the last year		Yes, during the last year

Table 4–4. Alcohol Use Disorders Identification Test (AUDIT) (*continued*)

Questions	0	1	2	3	4
10. Has a relative, friend, doctor, or other health care worker been concerned about your drinking or suggested that you cut down?	No		Yes, but not in the last year		Yes, during the last year

Note. The minimum score (for nondrinkers) is 0, and the maximum possible score is 40. A score of 8 is indicative of hazardous and harmful alcohol use and possibly of alcohol dependence. Scores of 8–15 indicate a medium level, and scores of 16 and above indicate a high level of alcohol problems.

Source. Reproduced with permission from Babor TF, Biddle-Higgins JC, Saunders JB, et al.: *AUDIT: The Alcohol Use Disorders Identification Test: Guidelines for Use in Primary Health Care* (WHO/MSD/MSB/01.6a). Geneva, Switzerland, World Health Organization Department of Mental Health and Substance Dependence, 2001. Copyright 2001, World Health Organization.

a 2-day history of paranoid, delusional behavior will not rule out abuse, because cocaine has a relatively short half-life (it clears in 24–36 hours) and because paper chromatography has a low sensitivity (Gold and Dackis 1986).
Marijuana, which is highly fat soluble, has a relatively long half-life and can
be detected in the urine of chronic heavy users up to 3 weeks after last use.
Most other substances are detectable in urine for only 2–3 days. It may be advisable to use many matrices (hair, oral fluid, sweat, and urine) to reduce the
success evaluees may have in attempting to cheat.

Urine Drug Screens

Urine drug screen results usually are reported as either positive or negative for
any particular drug. It is important to know the cutoff ranges the particular
test (or laboratory definition) identifies as "negative." Most routine urine
screens cover the major drugs of abuse. Specificity and sensitivity are lower
with thin-layer chromatography (TLC) and immunoassay techniques. More
sophisticated and sensitive quantitative testing with gas chromatography–
mass spectrometry (GC-MS) can be done later for certain drugs (e.g., marijuana) if urine from the original sample tests positive. Urine drug screen results are not typically useful in court because they do not answer the question
of degree of intoxication.

For general hospital purposes, urine drug screens are imperative in certain
situations. In coma of unknown etiology, in atypical psychiatric presentations, or in agitated and confused patients with known drug histories or with
physical evidence of substance abuse, urine drug screening should be routine.
For high-risk populations or in areas where drug abuse is epidemic (e.g., certain inner-city general hospitals), urine drug screening should be routinely
conducted for psychiatric admissions. To ensure the validity and reliability of
urine screen results, direct observation of voiding may be indicated. Finally,
it should be noted that morning urine samples are often contaminated; use of
morning samples for screening should be avoided if possible.

A new compound of interest is ethyl glucuronide (EtG), which is a metabolite of alcohol metabolism in the liver and which may be detected in urine.
The urine test for EtG is being used widely, as it has a high *sensitivity* and reflects hepatic metabolism of ethanol within 3–5 days. A great deal of caution
is needed in using this test because its *specificity* as a test of alcoholic beverages
is unknown. Its sensitivity provides that hundreds of household and personal

items may lead to a positive test result (even transdermal absorption of alcohol-based hand cleaners). In 2006, the Substance Abuse and Mental Health Services Administration published an advisory against reliance on this test as a singular measure of lapse or relapse, and the warning persists to this point.

Blood Screening Tests

Suspicion of alcohol or other substance abuse may be heightened with corroborating laboratory evidence from blood studies (Table 4–5), which is often useful in forensic cases. Blood studies showing elevated mean corpuscular volume (MCV) and liver function tests showing elevated aspartate transaminase (AST; formerly known as serum glutamic-oxaloacetic transaminase [SGOT]), alanine transaminase (ALT; formerly known as serum glutamic-pyruvic transaminase [SGPT]), and lactate dehydrogenase (LDH) may point to alcohol abuse. Elevated serum gamma-glutamyl transpeptidase (SGGT; a sensitive measure of liver enzyme induction) is an indicator of possible alcoholic liver disease. More than 70% of heavy drinkers have elevated SGGT levels (>40 units/L). Alcoholic individuals have a 4–10 times higher rate of abnormal SGGT levels when they are actively drinking than when they are abstinent. SGGT as a marker of heavy alcohol consumption has a sensitivity of 70% and a specificity of 90%. AST/SGOT is elevated (>45 units/L) in 30%–60% of alcoholics, with a sensitivity of 80%. Irwin et al. (1988) reported preliminary evidence that increases of 20% for SGGT levels and of 50% for AST/SGOT levels over baseline abstinence levels are possible markers of heavy drinking (even if the increased values fall within the normal range) and therefore may indicate relapse.

Elevated MCV, a measure of red blood cell size (>95 cubic microns in males, 100 in females), is found in certain nutritional deficiencies (e.g., folate, B_{12}) or can be associated with alcohol's direct effects on bone marrow cell production. Increased MCV is found in 45%–90% of alcoholics, whereas only 1%–5% of nonalcoholics demonstrate elevated MCV. The sensitivity of MCV in detecting heavy drinking is around 30%–50%; its specificity may be higher than 90%.

Attempts are being made to develop laboratory profiles that will serve as better markers for early detection of alcohol problems. For example, the combination of abnormal SGGT and MCV identifies 90% of alcoholics in the general medical population, compared with 70%–80% when MCV or

Table 4–5. Laboratory findings associated with alcohol abuse

Blood alcohol level

Positive Breathalyzer test

Elevated MCV

Elevated AST, ALT, LDH

Elevated SGGT (particularly sensitive)

Decreased albumin, B_{12}, folic acid

Increased uric acid, elevated amylase, and evidence of bone marrow suppression

Increased %CDT (but only in heavy, sustained use)

Note. AST = aspartate transaminase (formerly known as serum glutamic-oxaloacetic transaminase [SGOT]); ALT = alanine transaminase (formerly known as serum glutamic-pyruvic transaminase [SGPT]); CDT = carbohydrate-deficient transferrin; LDH = lactate dehydrogenase; MCV = mean corpuscular volume; SGGT = serum gamma-glutamyl transpeptidase.

SGGT is used alone (Lumeng 1986). Unfortunately, at this time, unacceptable rates of false-negative and false-positive results render these panels inappropriate for clinical applications other than screening. Other examples of markers for detection of substance abuse include decreased serum albumin, B_{12}, or folic acid, which may be evidence of prolonged malnutrition secondary to alcohol or substance abuse. Positive tests for hepatitis B, HIV, and bacteremia may indicate past or present intravenous use. Laboratory findings consistent with pancreatitis, hepatitis, bone marrow suppression, or certain types of infection may be clues to underlying alcoholism.

In coming years, measurement of percentage carbohydrate-deficient transferrin (referred to as %CDT) will become increasingly important in detecting relapse and recent heavy alcohol use. The usefulness of this test centers on the finding that the percentage of transferrin with a deficient carbohydrate content increases after at least 2 weeks of daily consumption of more than 60 g of alcohol. Elevated levels of CDT indicate heavy alcohol exposure. The %CDT test has a sensitivity of around 70%–80% and a specificity of up to 90%. The test is superior to SGGT in detecting or confirming chronic heavy alcohol use (Hock et al. 2005). There are a few disorders, such as inborn disorders of glycoprotein metabolism, that will cause an increased %CDT in about 1%–2% of the population, and very severe liver disease can also lead to false-positive results. The %CDT test can be used to monitor a return to substantial drinking, but its utility in situations of minimal changes or related to minimal intake is uncertain and poses a risk for misuse of the test. Not everyone is "a good %CDT responder/elevator" (i.e., %CDT reliably alters with alcohol exposure), which is why SGGT should be obtained as well.

Other Laboratory Studies

There is increasing experience with the use of other body tissue, such as sweat, hair, and saliva, as laboratory specimens to test for substance use; however, the clinical reliability of laboratory assays with these screening matrices remains unknown. Breathalyzer tests are simple and noninvasive, provide immediate results, and are widely used. Liver, spleen, and brain scans as well as electroencephalography may also be useful in the diagnosis of substance abuse. Imaging studies have been powerful tools in research on the neuroanatomic and neurochemical aspects of addiction, but their place in diagnosis or assessment (except in obvious cases of alcohol-induced cortical damage) is limited. Breath alcohol levels are less invasive, but their usefulness may be limited by an individual's poor lung capacity.

Tests of skin and hair are minimally invasive assessment tools. Hair testing is becoming increasingly popular as a way to test for both current and remote drug use. When drugs are present in the blood system, they are also present and stored in the hair follicle. Hair from any part of the body is acceptable for use in analysis. A new technology, a bracelet or anklet that constantly measures alcohol levels in the skin, may be available soon.

Interpretation of Laboratory Findings

Qualitative presence of drugs indicates prior exposure but perhaps not current intoxication or impairment. To get to the truth, consider the following points:

- What method was used?
- Did the assay analyze for the drug, the metabolite, or both?
- What is the cutoff threshold? (call the lab if unclear)
- Was the time of sampling close to the time of exposure?

Speaking to the laboratory that performs or manufactures the test can sometimes be helpful in elucidating confusing results.

False-Positive Results

When considering the possibility of a false-positive result, first ask whether a false positive is possible. A false-positive result from TLC is highly unlikely, because this method is highly specific, albeit poorly sensitive, both for drugs and for their metabolites and because color dyes increase specificity. In radio-immunoassay (RIA) or enzyme-multiplied immunoassay technique (EMIT), two sensitive tests, chemically similar compounds may cross-react, producing false positives. Furthermore, because each antibody has a particular affinity, the specificity of each test should be evaluated. Immunoassays can be confirmed by chromatography, and vice versa. It is also important to be aware that various prescription psychopharmacological agents can cause false positives. For example, bupropion can cause false-positive results on assays for amphetamine/methamphetamine, although not when GC-MS testing is done.

False-Negative Results

False negatives occur more easily than false positives. Remember that once a specimen tests negative, it is not further tested. Nonetheless, negative TLC results are not conclusive. Cutoffs may be too high for RIA or enzyme immunoassay (EIA). When suspicion for use is strong, the clinician should repeat the test and consult the laboratory for more sensitive drug-screening procedures such as GC-MS.

Urine Characteristics

Most urine drug screens will report a specific gravity as well as drug information. A low specific gravity indicates that the urine concentration is low and suggests that the evaluee could have ingested a large volume of fluid in order to dilute concentrations of the drug below the threshold needed for a positive test. Also, these tests usually include a way of assessing the approximate temperature of a sample. A sample that tests below body temperature could mean that the sample was diluted with something in the testing room, such as toilet water, or that it came from outside the body.

Imaging Studies

Various types of imaging studies are valuable in the treatment of substance use disorders, particularly in the assessment of associated conditions, such as alcohol-induced dementia, a cerebrovascular accident in the context of cocaine use, or chronic obstructive pulmonary disease in tobacco smoking. There are many research uses for imaging as well. However, at this time, imaging studies are not essential aspects of substance use disorder assessment.

Key Points

- Treatment is optimized by successful assessment and diagnosis.
- Be aware that what is considered a positive test result may depend on the specific hospital's or laboratory's rules.
- There are many reasons—clinical, employment, judicial—to screen for substances of abuse.
- Various methods are used to try to cheat on urine drug screens.
- Testing is as important as other parts of the clinical assessment.
- Test results indicating use do not necessarily indicate addiction or dependence.
- Be aware of the limitations of specific tests and when additional confirmatory tests are needed.

References

American Psychiatric Association: Diagnostic and Statistical Manual of Mental Disorders, 4th Edition. Washington, DC, American Psychiatric Association, 1994

Babor TF, Biddle-Higgins JC, Saunders JB, et al: AUDIT: The Alcohol Use Disorders Identification Test: Guidelines for Use in Primary Health Care (WHO/MSD/MSB/01.6a). Geneva, Switzerland, World Health Organization, 2001

Dawson DA, Das A, Faden VB, et al: Screening for high- and moderate-risk drinking during pregnancy: a comparison of several TWEAK-based screeners. Alcohol Clin Exp Res 25:1342–1349, 2001

Ewing JA: Detecting alcoholism: the CAGE Questionnaire. JAMA 252:1905–1907, 1984

Fudala PJ, Berkow, LC, Fralich JL, et al: Use of naloxone in the assessment of opioids dependence. Life Sci 49:1809–1814, 1991

Gold MS, Dackis CA: Role of the laboratory in the evaluation of suspected drug abuse. J Clin Psychiatry 47:17–23, 1986

Hock B, Schwarz M, Domke I, et al: Validity of carbohydrate-deficient transferrin (%CDT), gamma-glutamyltransferase (gamma-GT) and mean corpuscular erythrocyte volume (MCV) as biomarkers for chronic alcohol abuse: a study in patients with alcohol dependence and liver disorders of non-alcoholic and alcoholic origin. Addiction 100:1477–1486, 2005

Irwin M, Baird S, Smith TL, et al: Use of laboratory tests to monitor heavy drinking by alcoholic men discharged from a treatment program. Am J Psychiatry 145:595–599, 1988

Kaminer Y, Bukstein O, Tarter RE: The Teen-Addiction Severity Index: rationale and reliability. Int J Addiction 26:219–226, 1991

Kampman KM, Volpicelli JR, McGinnis DE, et al: Reliability and validity of the Cocaine Selective Severity Assessment. Addict Behav 23:449–461, 1998

Lumeng L: New diagnostic markers of alcohol abuse. Hepatology 6:742–745, 1986

MacAndrew C: The differentiation of male alcoholic outpatients from nonalcoholic outpatients by means of the MMPI. Q J Stud Alcohol 26:238–246, 1965

McLellan AT, Kushner H, Metzger D, et al: The Fifth Edition of the Addiction Severity Index. J Subst Abuse Treat 9:199–213, 1992

National Institute on Alcohol Abuse and Alcoholism: Helping Patients Who Drink Too Much: A Clinician's Guide, Updated 2005 Edition (NIH Publ No 07-3769). Bethesda, MD, National Institute on Alcohol Abuse and Alcoholism, January 2007

Reinert DF, Allen JP: The Alcohol Use Disorders Identification Test (AUDIT): a review of recent research. Alcohol Clin Exp Res 26:272–279, 2002

Rikoon SH, Cacciola JS, Carise D, et al: Predicting DSM-IV dependence diagnoses from Addiction Severity Index composite scores. J Subst Abuse Treat 31:17–24, 2006

Russell M: New assessment tools for drinking in pregnancy: T-ACE, TWEAK, and others. Alcohol Health and Research World 18:55–61, 1994

Selzer ML: The Michigan Alcoholism Screening Test: the quest for a new diagnostic instrument. Am J Psychiatry 127:1653–1658, 1971

Sledjeski EM, Dierker LC, Costello D, et al: Predictive variability of four nicotine dependence measures in a college sample. Drug Alcohol Depend 1:10–19, 2007

Substance Abuse and Mental Health Services Administration: The role of biomarkers in the treatment of alcohol use disorders (DHHS Publ No SMA 06-4223; NCADI Publ No MS996). Substance Abuse Treatment Advisory 5(4), September 2006

Sullivan JT, Sykora K, Schneiderman J, et al: Assessment of alcohol withdrawal: the revised Clinical Institute Withdrawal Assessment for Alcohol scale (CIWA-Ar). Br J Addict 84:1353–1357, 1989

Wesson DR, Ling W: The Clinical Opiate Withdrawal Scale (COWS). J Psychoactive Drugs 2:253–259, 2003

5

Definition, Presentation, and Diagnosis

Nosology

Advances in biological and psychosocial understanding of substance use disorders (SUDs) have informed an evolution of their classification concurrent with the development of operational criteria such as DSM-IV (American Psychiatric Association 1994) and its Text Revision, DSM-IV-TR (American Psychiatric Association 2000), and assessment instruments such as the Structured Clinical Interview for DSM-IV (SCID; Spitzer et al. 1995). DSM-IV-TR provides generic definitions of dependence, abuse, and withdrawal, as well as specific definitions for several substance-induced syndromes. Throughout this chapter we review all DSM drug categories with comments on some specific conditions for each substance.

DSM-IV Context

This chapter begins by reviewing some basic points about DSM's approach to substances of abuse.

1. In DSM-IV, the term *substance* can refer to a drug of abuse, a medication, or a toxin and need not be limited to agents that are "psychoactive."
2. The term *organic* is absent from DSM-IV. The disorders classified in DSM-III (American Psychiatric Association 1980) as substance-induced organic mental disorders were reclassified as SUDs in DSM-IV. DSM-IV distinguishes substance-induced mental disorders from those that are due to a general medical condition and those that have no specified etiology.
3. DSM-IV diagnoses require the presence of "clinically significant distress and impairment in social, occupational, or other important areas of functioning."
4. DSM-IV diagnoses require that the condition is not due to a general medical condition and is not better accounted for by another mental disorder.
5. DSM-IV-TR did not alter the definitions of mental disorders but instead provided updates to the descriptive text. The text notes that degree of tolerance may vary according to the specific substance's central nervous system (CNS) effects and that tolerance does occur in phenylcyclohexylpiperidine (phencyclidine [PCP]) use. DSM-IV-TR emphasizes the utility of laboratory tests, such as toxicology screens and serum gamma-glutamyltransferase (SGGT) assays, in detection of relapse (see Chapter 4, "Evaluation and Assessment").

Generic Definitions and Diagnosis

Substance Use Disorders

Substance Dependence

Dependence refers to a set of cognitive, behavioral, and physiological features that together signify continued use despite significant substance-related problems. It is a pattern of repeated self-administration that can result in tolerance, withdrawal, and compulsive drug-taking behavior. To qualify for a DSM-IV-

TR diagnosis of substance dependence, a patient must exhibit, over a 12-month period, three or more characteristics from a seven-item polythetic criteria set (Table 5–1). Neither tolerance nor withdrawal is necessary or sufficient for a diagnosis of substance dependence. However, a history of tolerance or withdrawal is usually associated with a more severe clinical course. Tolerance—the need for greatly increased amounts of a substance to produce a desired effect, or a greatly diminished effect with constant use of the same amount of the substance—may be difficult to discern from the patient's history when the substance used is of unknown purity. In such situations, quantitative laboratory tests may help. Withdrawal occurs when blood or tissue concentrations of a substance decline in an individual who had maintained prolonged heavy use of the substance. In this state, the person will likely take the substance to relieve or avoid unpleasant withdrawal symptoms.

According to DSM-IV-TR, remission may be noted as early full, early partial, sustained full, or sustained partial. The presence or absence of physiological dependence (i.e., evidence of tolerance or withdrawal), current use of agonist therapy, and placement in a controlled environment may also be specified.

Substance Abuse

In DSM-IV-TR, substance *abuse* refers to continued use despite significant problems caused by the use in those who do not meet criteria for substance dependence. "Failure to fulfill major role obligations" is a criterion. To fulfill a criterion, the substance-related problem must have occurred repeatedly or persistently during the same 12-month period. The criteria for abuse do not include tolerance, withdrawal, or compulsive use (Table 5–2). Substance abuse cannot be applied to use of caffeine and nicotine. The term *abuse* should not be used as a blanket term for *use, misuse,* or *hazardous use.*

Substance-Induced Disorders

Substance Intoxication

Substance *intoxication* (Table 5–3) is a reversible syndrome resulting from recent exposure to a substance. It is often associated, and may be concurrently diagnosed, with substance abuse or dependence. The category does not apply to nicotine. Different substances (sometimes, even different substance classes) may produce identical symptoms during intoxication.

Table 5–1.   DSM-IV-TR diagnostic criteria for substance dependence

A maladaptive pattern of substance use, leading to clinically significant impairment or distress, as manifested by three (or more) of the following, occurring at any time in the same 12-month period:

(1)   tolerance, as defined by either of the following:

    (a)   a need for markedly increased amounts of the substance to achieve intoxication or desired effect

    (b)   markedly diminished effect with continued use of the same amount of the substance

(2)   withdrawal, as manifested by either of the following:

    (a)   the characteristic withdrawal syndrome for the substance (refer to Criteria A and B of the criteria sets for withdrawal from the specific substances)

    (b)   the same (or a closely related) substance is taken to relieve or avoid withdrawal symptoms

(3)   the substance is often taken in larger amounts or over a longer period than was intended

(4)   there is a persistent desire or unsuccessful efforts to cut down or control substance use

(5)   a great deal of time is spent in activities necessary to obtain the substance (e.g., visiting multiple doctors or driving long distances), use the substance (e.g., chain-smoking), or recover from its effects

(6)   important social, occupational, or recreational activities are given up or reduced because of substance use

(7)   the substance use is continued despite knowledge of having a persistent or recurrent physical or psychological problem that is likely to have been caused or exacerbated by the substance (e.g., current cocaine use despite recognition of cocaine-induced depression, or continued drinking despite recognition that an ulcer was made worse by alcohol consumption)

Specify if:

With Physiological Dependence: evidence of tolerance or withdrawal (i.e., either item 1 or 2 is present)

Without Physiological Dependence: no evidence of tolerance or withdrawal (i.e., neither item 1 nor 2 is present)

Course specifiers (see text for definitions):

Early Full Remission
Early Partial Remission
Sustained Full Remission
Sustained Partial Remission
On Agonist Therapy
In a Controlled Environment

Table 5–2. DSM-IV-TR diagnostic criteria for substance abuse

A. A maladaptive pattern of substance use leading to clinically significant impairment or distress, as manifested by one (or more) of the following, occurring within a 12-month period:

   (1) recurrent substance use resulting in a failure to fulfill major role obligations at work, school, or home (e.g., repeated absences or poor work performance related to substance use; substance-related absences, suspensions, or expulsions from school; neglect of children or household)

   (2) recurrent substance use in situations in which it is physically hazardous (e.g., driving an automobile or operating a machine when impaired by substance use)

   (3) recurrent substance-related legal problems (e.g., arrests for substance-related disorderly conduct)

   (4) continued substance use despite having persistent or recurrent social or interpersonal problems caused or exacerbated by the effects of the substance (e.g., arguments with spouse about consequences of intoxication, physical fights)

B. The symptoms have never met the criteria for substance dependence for this class of substance.

Table 5–3. DSM-IV-TR diagnostic criteria for substance intoxication

A. The development of a reversible substance-specific syndrome due to recent ingestion of (or exposure to) a substance. **Note:** Different substances may produce similar or identical syndromes.

B. Clinically significant maladaptive behavioral or psychological changes that are due to the effect of the substance on the central nervous system (e.g., belligerence, mood lability, cognitive impairment, impaired judgment, impaired social or occupational functioning) and develop during or shortly after use of the substance.

C. The symptoms are not due to a general medical condition and are not better accounted for by another mental disorder.

Substance Withdrawal

Withdrawal (Table 5–4) is a behavioral, physiological, and cognitive state resulting from cessation of, or reduction in, heavy and prolonged substance use. Perhaps all withdrawing individuals crave the substance to reduce withdrawal

Table 5–4.   DSM-IV-TR diagnostic criteria for substance withdrawal

A.   The development of a substance-specific syndrome due to the cessation of (or reduction in) substance use that has been heavy and prolonged.

B.   The substance-specific syndrome causes clinically significant distress or impairment in social, occupational, or other important areas of functioning.

C.   The symptoms are not due to a general medical condition and are not better accounted for by another mental disorder.

symptoms. Signs and symptoms vary according to the substance used; most symptoms of withdrawal are the opposite of those observed in intoxication by the same substance. Withdrawal is usually associated with substance dependence.

Substance-Induced Mental Disorders

In DSM-IV-TR, the category Substance-Induced Mental Disorders Included Elsewhere in the Manual refers to conditions that include "a variety of symptoms that are characteristic of other mental disorders," such as primary psychotic, mood, or anxiety disorders. Among this group, three substance-induced disorders are termed "persisting": substance-induced persisting dementia, substance-induced persisting amnestic disorder (which applies to various substances), and hallucinogen persisting perception disorder (flashbacks). The various substance-induced mental disorders are classified among the disorders with which they share psychopathology (e.g., cannabis-induced psychotic disorder is included in the Schizophrenia and Other Psychotic Disorders section). Context specifiers are provided with which one may indicate whether the disorder began during intoxication or during withdrawal from the substance. Diagnosis of a substance-induced mental disorder requires evidence of intoxication or withdrawal. Some disorders can persist after the substance has been eliminated from the body, but symptoms lasting more than 4 weeks after acute intoxication or withdrawal are considered manifestations either of a primary mental disorder or a substance-induced persisting disorder. This differential diagnosis is complicated: withdrawal from some substances (e.g., sedatives) may partially mimic intoxication with others (e.g., amphetamines). The fact that a syndrome (e.g., depression with suicidal ideation) is caused by a substance (e.g., cocaine) in no way diminishes its clinical import. In most cases, intoxication and withdrawal are distinguished from the substance-induced disorders of the same class because the symptoms in these latter disorders are in excess of those usually associated with intoxication with or withdrawal from that substance and are severe enough to warrant independent clinical attention.

Alcohol

Alcohol Use Disorders

Although some groups have referred to alcohol dependence as "alcoholism," the term has had no operational definition. It is important to distinguish *abuse* from *dependence,* because whereas the individual who abuses alcohol has some chance of drinking in a controlled manner, someone who is dependent has no choice but to become abstinent. Of course, it is difficult to predict which persons who abuse alcohol will go on to dependence. Even among persons whose drinking can be characterized as alcohol abuse, a goal of abstinence is safer and prevents progression to dependence.

Alcohol Dependence

The DSM-IV-TR diagnostic criteria for alcohol dependence follow those for other substance disorders, as delineated in Table 5–1. The presence of physiological dependence has prognostic value, because it indicates a more severe clinical course, perhaps more so for alcohol withdrawal than for tolerance (De Bruijn et al. 2005).

Alcohol Abuse

Fewer symptoms are required for a diagnosis of alcohol abuse than for dependence, and alcohol abuse is diagnosed only after dependence has been ruled out. Drinking when driving and (for a physician) drinking before seeing patients are two examples of use of alcohol when a person is expected to fulfill role obligations. The development of medical and psychiatric complications related to alcohol use may aid in diagnosis.

Alcohol-Induced Disorders

Alcohol Intoxication

Alcohol intoxication is time-limited and reversible, with onset depending on tolerance, amount ingested, and amount absorbed. It is affected by interactions with other substances, medical status, and individual variation. Table 5–5 lists blood alcohol levels (BALs) and corresponding clinical features of a nonhabituated patient. For the habituated patient, the presentation can vary greatly. Intoxication stages range from mild inebriation to anesthesia, coma, respiratory depression, and death. Relative to degree of tolerance, increasing BALs can lead to euphoria, mild coordination problems, ataxia, confusion, and decreased consciousness; BALs greater than 0.4 mg% can result in anesthesia, coma, and death. However, chronic heavy drinkers maintain high BALs with fewer effects. Alcohol intoxication may affect heart rate and electroencephalogram (EEG) readings and may cause nystagmus, slow reaction times, and behavioral changes, including mood lability, impaired judgment, impaired social or occupational functioning, cognitive problems, and disinhibition of sexual or aggressive impulses. Intoxication with alcohol closely resembles sedative, hypnotic, or anxiolytic intoxication. Individual and cultural variations of tolerance may influence symptom presentation. Other neurological conditions such as cerebellar ataxia from multiple sclerosis may mimic some of the physiological signs and symptoms of alcohol intoxication. "Alcohol idiosyncratic intoxication" is not present in DSM-IV-TR, but could be diagnosed as alcohol use disorder not otherwise specified. It should be noted that the odor of alcohol should not discount the possibility that more than one substance is being used.

Alcohol Withdrawal

Any relative drop in BAL can precipitate withdrawal, even during continuous alcohol consumption. Features include the following symptoms: coarse tremor of hands, tongue, or eyelids; nausea or vomiting; malaise or weakness; autonomic hyperactivity; orthostatic hypotension; anxiety; depressed mood; irritability; transient hallucinations (generally poorly formed) or illusions; headache; and insomnia. The generalized tremor, which is coarse and of fast frequency (5–7 Hz), can worsen with motor activity or emotional stress; it is most likely to be observed on extension of the hands or tongue. Often, pa-

Table 5–5. Blood alcohol level (BAL) and typical clinical presentation in the nontolerant, alcohol-intoxicated patient

BAL (mg/dL)	Clinical presentation
30	Attention difficulties (mild), euphoria
50	Coordination problems; driving is legally impaired
100	Ataxia, drunk driving
200	Confusion, decreased consciousness
>400	Anesthesia, ?coma, ?death

Note. ? = possible.

tients complain only of feeling shaky inside. Careful attention should be paid to vital signs in a suspected alcoholic. Symptoms peak 24–48 hours after the last drink and subside in 5–7 days, even without treatment. Insomnia and irritability may last 10 days or longer. The withdrawal symptoms may precipitate a relapse. Complications of major motor seizures ("rum fits") occur and are more likely to develop in those with a history of epilepsy and in those with other medical illnesses, malnutrition, fatigue, and depression.

Other Alcohol-Induced Disorders

Alcohol Intoxication or Withdrawal Delirium

Delirium tremens (DTs) can result from alcohol withdrawal or intoxication. It differs from uncomplicated withdrawal in that the delirium may include abnormal perceptions, agitation, terror, insomnia, mild fever, or autonomic instability. Hallucinations may be auditory and of a persecutory nature, or they may be kinesthetic, such as tactile sensations of crawling insects. Yet, a wide variation of presentations can occur, from quiet confusion, agitation, and peculiar behavior lasting several weeks to marked abnormal behavior, vivid, terrifying delusions, and other disorders of perception. DTs can appear suddenly but usually occurs gradually, 2–3 days after cessation of drinking, with peak intensity on day 4 or day 5. DTs is usually benign and short-lived. The majority of cases subside after 3 days; subacute symptoms may last 4–5 weeks. Although early reports noted that up to 20% of cases may end fatally, later reports indicate that the fatality rate may be less than 1%. DTs is associated with infections, subdural hematomas, trauma, liver disease, and metabolic disorders, and the cause of death is usually infectious fat emboli or cardiac arrhythmias (usually associated with hyperkalemia, hyperpyrexia, and poor hydration). DTs generally occurs in withdrawing alcoholics with 5–15 years of heavy drinking.

Alcohol Withdrawal Seizures

Alcohol withdrawal seizures that are not a part of DTs generally occur 7–38 hours (usually about 24 hours) after last alcohol use in chronic drinkers. Half of these occur in bursts of two to six grand mal seizures. Fewer than 3% of patients in withdrawal develop status epilepticus. A total of 10% of all chronic drinkers experience a grand mal seizure, one-third of all who seize progress to DTs, and one-fiftieth of all who seize go on to status epilepticus. Focal seizures suggest a focal lesion, which may indicate trauma or epilepsy. Hypomagnesemia, respiratory alkalosis, hypoglycemia, and increased intracellular sodium have all been associated with these seizures. Serum magnesium levels should be obtained in alcoholic patients who develop seizures. Alcohol withdrawal seizures have important prognostic value in predicting a complicated withdrawal period.

Alcohol-Induced Persisting Dementia

Prolonged and heavy use of alcohol may be followed by dementia. Diagnosis is confirmed by its presence at least 3 weeks after ending alcohol intake. In this condition, unlike alcohol-induced amnestic disorder, cognitive impairment affects more than memory function and no cause other than alcohol is found.

Alcohol-Induced Persisting Amnestic Disorder (Korsakoff's Syndrome)

Thiamine (vitamin B_1) deficiency associated with prolonged heavy use of alcohol produces this amnesia and its associated neurological deficits (peripheral neuropathy, cerebellar ataxia, and myopathy). It often follows acute Wernicke's encephalopathy (confusion, ataxia, nystagmus, ophthalmoplegia, and other neurological signs). As Wernicke's encephalopathy subsides, severe impairment of anterograde and retrograde memory remains; confabulation is common. Early treatment of Wernicke's encephalopathy with large doses of thiamine may prevent Korsakoff's syndrome. Unlike other dementias, Korsakoff's syndrome is characterized by preserved intellectual function.

Alcohol-Induced Psychotic Disorder With Delusions or Hallucinations

Alcohol-induced psychotic disorder with hallucinations is far more common than alcohol-induced psychotic disorder with delusions. The hallucinosis manifests as vivid and persistent hallucinations, usually within 48 hours after reduction of alcohol in dependent patients. Auditory or visual hallucinations can occur. This disorder may last several weeks or months. Hallucinations may range from sounds (e.g., clicks, roaring, humming, ringing bells, chanting) to threatening or derogatory voices. One derogatory remark may engender relentlessly persisting auditory accusations and commands by several voices. Patients usually respond with fear, anxiety, and agitation. Diagnosis is usually based on a history of heavy alcohol use, lack of formal thought disorder, and lack of psychosis in the personal or family history. In the majority of cases, the symptoms recede in a few hours to days, with the patients fully realizing the perceptions were imaginary. Rarely, patients develop a quiet chronic paranoid delusional state indistinguishable from frank schizophrenia, from which remission would not be expected after 6 months. Overall, differential diagnosis includes DTs, withdrawal syndrome, paranoid psychosis, and borderline transient psychotic episodes. In contrast to DTs, these hallucinations usually occur in a clear consciousness. Lack of autonomic symptoms differentiates the syndrome from withdrawal.

Alcohol-Induced Sexual Dysfunction

Alcohol broadly affects reproductive function, generally in proportion to the magnitude of use. Contrary to myth, both men and women have decreased sexual function when they are alcohol dependent.

Blackouts

Blackouts are periods of amnesia during periods of intoxication (by most CNS depressants) despite a state of consciousness that seems normal. They may occur in nonalcoholics during heavy drinking or at any time during alcohol dependence. Severity and duration of use correlate with blackout occurrence.

Sedatives, Hypnotics, and Anxiolytics

The sedative, hypnotic, and anxiolytic substances include the benzodiazepines, the selective nonbenzodiazepine hypnotics (e.g., zaleplon and zolpidem, which act at the benzodiazepine receptor and are reinforcing to recovering addicts), the carbamates (e.g., meprobamate), the barbiturates (e.g., secobarbital), and the barbiturate-like hypnotics (e.g., methaqualone). The sedative, hypnotic, and anxiolytic class includes all prescription sleeping medications (e.g., chloral hydrate, paraldehyde) and almost all prescription anxiolytics. The nonbenzodiazepine anxiolytics (e.g., buspirone, gepirone) are not included. Polysubstance abusers frequently self-medicate with sedatives to treat undesirable effects of cocaine or amphetamine. Definitions for this class and other classes of drugs follow the generic definitions of dependence and abuse presented in Tables 5–1 and 5–2. This class of substances produces secondary clinical syndromes that generally parallel those of alcohol, but their pharmacokinetics differ from alcohol in important ways. It is important to distinguish legitimate use of these medications from adaptation and maladaptive habituation, and from illegal use.

Sedative, Hypnotic, or Anxiolytic Use Disorders

Sedative, Hypnotic, or Anxiolytic Dependence

A diagnosis of dependence on sedatives, hypnotics, or anxiolytics should be considered only when, in addition to having physiological dependence, the individual using the substance shows evidence of a range of problems (e.g., an individual who has developed drug-seeking behavior to the extent that important activities are given up or reduced to obtain the substance). In this class of drugs, degree of physical dependence is closely related to dosage and length of use. For example, an individual who has taken benzodiazepines for long periods of time at prescribed and therapeutic doses and abruptly discontinues use may show signs of tolerance and withdrawal in the absence of a diagnosis of substance dependence.

Sedative-, Hypnotic-, or Anxiolytic-Induced Disorders

Sedative, Hypnotic, or Anxiolytic Intoxication

Memory impairment, which can be quite disturbing to the individual, is a prominent feature of sedative, hypnotic, or anxiolytic intoxication and is most often characterized by an anterograde amnesia that resembles alcoholic blackouts. As with other CNS depressants, one (or more) of the following signs develop during, or shortly after, sedative, hypnotic, or anxiolytic use: slurred speech, incoordination, unsteady gait, nystagmus, impairment in attention or memory, stupor, and coma.

Sedative, Hypnotic, or Anxiolytic Withdrawal

Sedative, hypnotic, or anxiolytic withdrawal is a characteristic syndrome that develops after a decrease in intake after regular use. Even a low dose of diazepam (5–10 mg) over time can result in significant withdrawal on abrupt cessation. Benzodiazepine abuse can involve several hundred milligrams of diazepam or its equivalent. Individuals who tolerate such dosages are dependent and require active substance abuse treatment with medications. As with alcohol, benzodiazepine withdrawal includes two or more symptoms such as autonomic hyperactivity, tremor, insomnia, anxiety, nausea, vomiting, and psychomotor agitation.

Relief on administration of any sedative-hypnotic agent supports a diagnosis of withdrawal. Grand mal seizures occur in 20%–30% of untreated individuals. The withdrawal syndrome produced by substances in this class may present as a life-threatening delirium. In severe withdrawal, perceptual disturbances can occur (if the person's reality testing is intact and sensorium clear, the specifier "with perceptual disturbances" should be noted). The timing and severity of the syndrome depend on the pharmacokinetics and pharmacodynamics of the substance. For drugs with longer half-lives, symptoms may develop more slowly than for those with shorter half-lives. There may be additional longer-term symptoms at a much lower level of intensity that persist for several months. As with alcohol, lingering withdrawal symptoms (e.g., anxiety, moodiness, and trouble sleeping) can be mistaken for non-substance-induced anxiety or depressive disorders (e.g., generalized anxiety disorder).

Sedative, Hypnotic, or Anxiolytic Withdrawal Delirium

Sedative, hypnotic, or anxiolytic withdrawal delirium is characterized by disturbances in consciousness and cognition, with visual, tactile, or auditory hallucinations. When present, withdrawal delirium should be diagnosed instead of withdrawal.

Opioids

Opioid Use Disorders

Opioid Dependence

Most individuals with opioid dependence have significant tolerance and experience withdrawal on abrupt discontinuation. The diagnosis requires the presence of features that reflect compulsive use without legitimate medical purpose or use of doses that are greatly in excess of that needed for pain relief.

Opioid Abuse

Dependence, rather than abuse, should be considered when problems related to opioid use are accompanied by evidence of tolerance, withdrawal, or compulsive behavior related to the use of opioids.

Opioid-Induced Disorders

Opioids are less likely than most other drugs of abuse to produce psychiatric symptoms and may reduce such symptoms. Opioid intoxication and opioid withdrawal are distinguished from the other opioid-induced disorders because the symptoms in these latter disorders are in excess of those usually associated with intoxication or withdrawal and are severe enough to warrant independent clinical attention.

Opioid Intoxication

The magnitude of the behavioral and physiological changes that result from opioid use depends on the dose as well as characteristics of the user. Symptoms of intoxication usually last as long as the half-life of the drug. Intoxication is marked by miosis or, if severe, by mydriasis (due to anoxia). Drowsiness, slurred speech, and impairment in attention and memory are other signs. Aggression and violence are rarely seen. When hallucinations occur in the absence of intact reality testing, a diagnosis of *opioid-induced psychotic disorder, with hallucinations* should be considered. Intoxication by alcohol, sedatives, hypnotics, or anxiolytics resembles opioid intoxication but does not produce miosis or a response to a naloxone (Narcan) challenge.

Opioid overdose is an emergency that can be diagnosed quickly; it manifests as coma, shock, pinpoint pupils (pupil dilation in severe cases), and depressed respiration, which may lead to death. It rapidly responds to naloxone, an opioid receptor antagonist; a lack of response to naloxone undermines a presumed diagnosis of opioid overdose. However, if other classes of drugs are responsible for the altered mental state, naloxone will produce only partial improvement. Opioid intoxication can be distinguished from alcohol and sedative intoxication by the presence of pupillary constriction and by toxicological testing. Precipitation of opioid overdose through ingestion of combinations of substances including alcohol, benzodiazepines, and barbiturates is a common complication and cause of death for those using high doses.

Opioid Withdrawal

Opioid withdrawal (Table 5–6) is a syndrome that follows a relative reduction in heavy and prolonged use. The syndrome begins within 6–8 hours after the last dose and peaks at 48–72 hours; symptoms disappear in 7–10 days. The signs and symptoms of opioid withdrawal are opposite to the acute agonist effects: lacrimation, rhinorrhea, pupillary dilation, piloerection, diaphoresis, diarrhea, yawning, mild hypertension, tachycardia, fever, and insomnia. A flu-like syndrome comes with complaints, demands, and drug seeking. Although intense, uncomplicated withdrawal usually is not life-threatening unless there is a severe underlying disorder, such as cardiac disease. The anxiety and restlessness associated with opioid withdrawal resemble symptoms seen in sedative, hypnotic, or anxiolytic withdrawal. However, opioid withdrawal is also accompanied by rhinorrhea, lacrimation, and mydriasis, which are not seen in sedative-type withdrawal.

Cocaine

Cocaine can be administered using coca leaves (chewed), coca paste (smoked), cocaine hydrochloride powder (inhaled or injected), and cocaine alkaloid (freebase or crack) (smoked). "Speedballing"—mixing cocaine and heroin—is

Table 5–6.   DSM-IV-TR diagnostic criteria for opioid withdrawal

A. Either of the following:

    (1) cessation of (or reduction in) opioid use that has been heavy and prolonged (several weeks or longer)

    (2) administration of an opioid antagonist after a period of opioid use

B. Three (or more) of the following, developing within minutes to several days after Criterion A:

    (1) dysphoric mood

    (2) nausea or vomiting

    (3) muscle aches

    (4) lacrimation or rhinorrhea

    (5) pupillary dilation, piloerection, or sweating

    (6) diarrhea

    (7) yawning

    (8) fever

    (9) insomnia

C. The symptoms in Criterion B cause clinically significant distress or impairment in social, occupational, or other important areas of functioning.

D. The symptoms are not due to a general medical condition and are not better accounted for by another mental disorder.

particularly dangerous due to potentiation of respiratory depressant effects. Cocaine-induced states should be distinguished from the symptoms of schizophrenia (paranoid type), bipolar and other mood disorders, generalized anxiety disorder, and panic disorder.

Cocaine Use Disorders

Cocaine Dependence

Exposure to cocaine can quickly produce dependence. An early sign is a growing difficulty to resist the drug. With its short half-life, frequent use is needed to stay "high." Complications of chronic use are common and include paranoia, aggression, anxiety, depression, and weight loss. Tolerance occurs with repeated use (by any route of administration). Withdrawal symptoms, particularly dysphoria, can be seen but are usually transitory and associated with high-dose use.

Cocaine Abuse

The intensity and frequency of cocaine use are less for abuse than for dependence. Episodes of clinically significant use often occur around paydays or special occasions, leading to a pattern of brief periods (hours to days) of heavy use and longer periods (weeks to months) of nonsignificant use or abstinence. Dependence, rather than abuse, should be considered when tolerance, withdrawal, or compulsive behavior related to obtaining and using the drug accompany use.

Cocaine-Induced Disorders

Cocaine Intoxication

Cocaine intoxication is a state that develops during, or shortly after, cocaine use. After an initial high, cocaine intoxication produces one or more of the following effects: euphoria with enhanced vigor, gregariousness, hyperactivity, restlessness, hypervigilance, interpersonal sensitivity, talkativeness, anxiety, tension, alertness, grandiosity, stereotyped and repetitive behavior, anger, and impaired judgment, and in the case of chronic intoxication, affective blunting with fatigue or sadness and social withdrawal. These features occur with two or more of the following: tachycardia or bradycardia; pupillary dilation; elevated or lowered blood pressure; perspiration or chills; nausea or vomiting; weight loss; psychomotor agitation or retardation; muscular weakness, respiratory depression, chest pain, or cardiac arrhythmias; and confusion, seizures, dyskinesias, dystonias, or coma. Cocaine's stimulant effects such as euphoria, tachycardia, hypertension, and psychomotor activity are more commonly seen than its depressant effects (sadness, bradycardia, hypotension, and psychomotor retardation), which emerge only with chronic high-dose use. Binges are highly reinforcing and may lead to psychosis or death. Cocaine's effects on the noradrenergic system are significant and in the overdose setting are associated with muscular twitching, rhabdomyolysis, seizures, cerebrovascular accidents, myocardial infarctions, arrhythmias, and respiratory failure.

Intravenous or freebase administration of cocaine greatly intensifies the rush, and use of this form can accelerate the progression to cocaine dependence. The half-life of cocaine used intravenously is less than 90 minutes, with euphoric effects lasting 15–20 minutes. Most cocaine is hydrolyzed to benzoylecgonine, which may be detected in the urine for up to 36 hours.

Metabolism is slowed when cocaine is combined with alcohol (forming coca-ethylene), in which case there is an 18- to 25-fold greater chance of death compared with cocaine alone. Smoked freebase has an onset of intense euphoria within seconds because it passes directly from the lungs to the systemic circulation. Euphoric effects depend on concentration and on the slope of the peak concentration (Schnoll 2005).

Tolerance to the euphoric effects develops during a binge; however, there is less tolerance for adverse experiences such as increasing anxiety, panic, or frank delirium. With prolonged cocaine administration, a transient delusional psychosis simulating paranoid schizophrenia can be seen. Usually the symptoms remit, although heavy, prolonged use or predisposing psychopathology may lead to persisting psychosis. Generally, higher dosages differentiate overdose from intoxication. Often, amphetamine or PCP intoxication can be distinguished from cocaine intoxication only by toxicological studies.

Cocaine Withdrawal

Cocaine withdrawal is accompanied by dysphoric mood, irritability, anxiety, fatigue, insomnia or hyposomnia, vivid and unpleasant dreams, and psychomotor agitation. Anhedonia and drug craving may be present. Withdrawal occurs more than 24 hours after cessation of use and generally peaks in 2–4 days (but irritability and depression may continue for months). Acute withdrawal symptoms are often seen after periods of repetitive high-dose use. These periods are characterized by intense and unpleasant feelings of lassitude and depression, perhaps with suicidal ideation, and generally require days of rest and recuperation. EEG abnormalities may be present.

Other Cocaine-Induced Disorders

Cocaine Intoxication Delirium

Cocaine intoxication delirium may occur within 24 hours of use. It may involve tactile and olfactory hallucinations, although violent or aggressive behavior is more frequent. Intoxication delirium is self-limited and usually resolves after 6 hours.

Cocaine-Induced Psychotic Disorder With Delusions

Cocaine-induced psychotic disorder with delusions is marked by rapidly developing persecutory delusions that may be accompanied by body image distortion, misperception of people's faces, formication, and aggression or violence.

Amphetamines

The amphetamine class includes substances with a substituted-phenylethyl-amine structure (e.g., amphetamine, dextroamphetamine, and methamphet-amine ["speed"]) and those that have amphetamine-like action but are structurally different (e.g., methylphenidate and most agents used as appetite suppressants). Signs and symptoms of amphetamine use parallel those of co-caine use, although effects may last longer. Amphetamine psychosis can resem-ble acute paranoid schizophrenia and frequently includes visual hallucinations. Patterns of use involve predominantly oral administration in pill form and re-semble those of cocaine use, with binge episodes alternating with crash symp-toms. Peripheral sympathomimetic effects may be quite potent.

Amphetamine-Induced Disorders

Amphetamine Intoxication

Amphetamine intoxication follows use of amphetamine or a related sub-stance. Behavioral and psychological changes are accompanied by at least two of the following: tachycardia or bradycardia, mydriasis, hypertension or hy-potension, perspiration or chills, nausea or vomiting, weight loss, psychomo-tor agitation or retardation, muscular weakness, respiratory depression, and chest pain. Confusion, arrhythmias, seizures, dyskinesias, dystonias, or coma may follow. The state begins no more than 1 hour after use, depending on the drug and method of delivery. "With perceptual disturbances" should be spec-ified when hallucinations or illusions occur in the absence of a delirium and with intact reality testing. If such disturbances occur in the absence of reality testing, a diagnosis of *amphetamine-induced psychotic disorder, with hallucina-tions* should be considered.

Differential Diagnosis of Amphetamine-Induced Disorders

Amphetamine-induced disorders may resemble primary mental disorders. Differentiating between amphetamine-induced psychosis and schizophrenia is very difficult (Caton et al. 2005). Intoxication by cocaine, hallucinogens, and PCP may cause a similar picture and can sometimes be distinguished from amphetamine intoxication only by urine or serum toxicology, although mydriasis, history of recent drug use, and speed of onset can be giveaways. Dependence on or abuse of amphetamines should be distinguished from cocaine, PCP, and hallucinogens dependence or abuse.

Phencyclidine and Ketamine

Originally an anesthetic, PCP ("angel dust," "PeaCe Pill") has become a street drug; its use in some urban areas is epidemic. Variations include ketamine (Ketalar) and the thiophene analogue of PCP, 1-[1-(2-thienyl)cyclohexyl]-piperidine (TCP). These substances can be used orally or intravenously and can be smoked and inhaled. PCP is often mixed with other substances such as amphetamines, cannabis, cocaine, or hallucinogens.

Phencyclidine Use Disorders

Phencyclidine Dependence

Dependence may have a rapid onset, and effects are generally unpredictable. The DSM-IV-TR diagnostic criteria for PCP dependence include the first seven items of generic definition of substance dependence, but Criteria 2a and 2b may not apply, given that a clear-cut withdrawal pattern is difficult to establish. As with hallucinogens, adverse reactions to PCP may be more common among individuals with preexisting mental disorders.

Phencyclidine Abuse

Individuals who abuse PCP may fail to fulfill role obligations because of intoxication. They may use in situations where it is physically hazardous. Recurrent social or interpersonal problems may result from the individual's intoxicated behavior or chaotic lifestyle, legal problems, or arguments with significant others.

Phencyclidine-Induced Disorders

Phencyclidine Intoxication

PCP intoxication begins after 5 minutes and peaks in 30 minutes. It produces affective instability, stereotypies, bizarre aggression, altered perception, disorganization, and confusion. Signs include hypertension, numbness, muscular rigidity, ataxia, and, at high dosages, hyperthermia and involuntary movements, followed by amnesia and coma, analgesia, seizures, and respiratory depression at the highest doses (greater than 20 mg). Milder intoxication resolves after 8–20 hours, but because of PCP's fat solubility, low-level intoxication may persist for many days. Mydriasis and nystagmus (vertical more often than horizontal) are characteristic of PCP use and help confirm diagnosis. The specifier "with perceptual disturbances" should be used if these signs are present.

Phencyclidine-Induced Psychotic Disorder

The most common PCP-induced disorder, PCP-induced psychotic disorder may occur in predisposed individuals. It may be indistinguishable from a psychotic episode. Chronic psychosis may occur, along with long-term neuropsychological deficits.

Differential Diagnosis of Phencyclidine-Induced Disorders

PCP-induced disorders may resemble primary mental disorders. Recurring episodes of psychotic or mood symptoms due to PCP may mimic schizophrenia or mood disorders. The fact of PCP use establishes a role for the substance in producing a mentally disordered state but does not rule out the co-occurrence of other primary mental disorders. And, although rapid onset of symptoms also suggests PCP use rather than a mental disorder, it may be that PCP use induces syndromes in individuals with preexisting disease. The course and the absence of a history of the disorder may aid in making this differentiation. Drug-related violence or impaired judgment may co-occur with, or may mimic aspects of, conduct disorder or antisocial personality disorder. Again, a history of disordered conduct may help to clarify the distinction. PCP users often use other drugs; thus, comorbid abuse of or dependence on other substances must be considered.

Hallucinogens

Hallucinogens are a diverse group of substances that include indolealkylamine derivatives (e.g., lysergic acid diethylamide [LSD], morning glory seeds), phenylalkylamine derivatives (e.g., mescaline, 2,5-dimethoxy-4-methylamphetamine [DOM or STP]), ring-substituted amphetamines (e.g.,

3,4-methylenedioxyamphetamine [MDA; "old" Ecstasy], 3,4-methylene-dioxymethamphetamine [MDMA; "new" Ecstasy]), 3,4-methylenedioxy-*N*-ethylamphetamine [MDEA]), indole alkaloids (e.g., psilocybin, dimethyltryptamine [DMT]), and miscellaneous other compounds. Excluded from this group are PCP, cannabis, and delta-9-tetrahydrocannabinol (THC). Hallucinogens are usually taken orally, although DMT is smoked, and use by injection does occur.

Hallucinogen Use Disorders

Hallucinogen Dependence

There are no specific criteria for hallucinogen dependence, and some of the generic dependence criteria do not apply, whereas others require qualification. Hallucinogen use is often limited to only a few times a week, even among individuals meeting full criteria for dependence. Tolerance to the euphoric and psychedelic effects of hallucinogens develops rapidly, but not to the autonomic effects (mydriasis, hyperreflexia, hypertension, increased body temperature, piloerection, and tachycardia). Cross-tolerance exists between LSD and other hallucinogens (e.g., psilocybin, mescaline). Withdrawal has not been demonstrated, although clear reports of "craving" after stopping hallucinogens are known. Some MDMA users describe a "hangover" the day after use that includes insomnia, fatigue, drowsiness, sore jaw muscles from teeth clenching, loss of balance, and headaches. Some of the reported adverse effects may be due to adulterant or substitute substances such as strychnine, PCP, or amphetamine.

Hallucinogen-Induced Disorders

Hallucinogen Intoxication

In hallucinogen intoxication perceptual changes occur alongside full alertness during or shortly after hallucinogen use. These changes include subjective intensification of perceptions, depersonalization, derealization, illusions, hallucinations, and synesthesias. DSM-IV-TR requires the presence of two of the given physiological signs. At low doses, the perceptual changes that occur often do not include hallucinations. Synesthesias (a blending of senses) may result in sounds being "seen." Hallucinations are usually visual, often of geometric forms, sometimes of persons and objects. Auditory or tactile hallucinations are rare. Reality testing is usually preserved. Intoxication should be differentiated from amphetamine or PCP intoxication. Toxicological tests help to make this differential. Intoxication with anticholinergics (e.g., trihexyphenidyl) can produce hallucinations, but they are often associated with fever, dry mouth and skin, flushed face, and visual disturbances.

Hallucinogen-Induced Psychotic Disorder

Hallucinogen-induced psychotic disorder may be brief or may lead into a long-lasting psychotic episode that is difficult to distinguish from schizophreniform disorder.

Hallucinogen Persisting Perception Disorder (Flashbacks)

Hallucinogen persisting perception disorder (flashbacks) following cessation of hallucinogen use is the reexperiencing of one or more of the same perceptual symptoms experienced while originally intoxicated. It is usually fleeting but in rare cases may be more lasting and persistent. It may be marked by noticing "trails" of moving objects, intensified flashes of colors, auditory and visual hallucinations, and false perceptions of movement. Symptoms may be triggered by stress, drug use (including that of other drugs such as cannabis), emergence into a dark environment, or even by intention. If the person's interpretation of the etiology of the state is delusional, the diagnosis is psychotic disorder not otherwise specified. Hallucinogen intoxication is distinguished from persisting perception disorder by temporal relation to use. Also, in posthallucinogen perception disorder, the individual does not believe that the perception represents external reality, whereas a person with a psychotic disorder often believes that the perception is real. Hallucinogen persisting perception disorder may be distinguished from migraine, epilepsy, or a neurological condition by neuro-ophthalmological history, physical examination, and appropriate laboratory evaluation.

Cannabis

The most commonly used substances in this class are marijuana, hashish, and purified THC. Usually smoked, these substances may also be mixed with food and eaten.

Cannabis Use Disorders

Cannabis Dependence

Dependence is marked by daily, or almost daily, compulsive cannabis use. Tolerance to most of the effects of cannabis has been reported in chronic users, but these patients do not generally develop physiological dependence, and such dependence is not a criterion for diagnosis in DSM-IV-TR. It should be noted, however, that although DSM-IV-TR does not include the diagnosis of cannabis withdrawal, there is a solid basis on which to describe a clinically significant withdrawal syndrome following heavy cannabis use (Budney and Hughes 2006).

Cannabis Abuse

Abuse is characterized by episodic use with maladaptive behavior. When significant levels of tolerance are present, or when psychological or physical problems are associated with cannabis in the context of compulsive use, dependence should be considered rather than abuse.

Cannabis-Induced Disorders

Cannabis Intoxication

Cannabis intoxication includes effects of the drug that are determined in major ways by the interaction of drug, person, and setting (route of administration, pharmacodynamics, and pharmacokinetics). Intoxication after smoking cannabis peaks after 10–30 minutes and lasts about 3 hours; metabolites may have a half-life of approximately 50 hours. Because most cannabinoids are fat soluble, their effects may occasionally persist or reoccur for 12–24 hours due to a slow release from fatty tissue or to enterohepatic circulation. Intoxication includes euphoria, anxiety, suspiciousness or paranoid ideation, sensation of slowed time, impaired judgment, and social withdrawal. Inappropriate laughter, panic attacks, and dysphoric affect may occur. Adverse reactions may be more common in those with psychiatric disorders or those frightened about the drug-taking situation. At least two of the following signs develop within 2 hours of use: 1) conjunctival injection, 2) increased appetite, 3) dry mouth, and 4) tachycardia. For differentiation, note that intoxication by alcohol or a sedative, hypnotic, or anxiolytic substance usually decreases appetite, increases aggressive behavior, and produces nystagmus or ataxia. In low doses, hallucinogens may cause symptoms that resemble cannabis intoxication. PCP intoxication is much more likely than cannabis intoxication to cause ataxia and aggressive behavior. DSM-IV-TR provides a specifier for cannabis intoxication with perceptual disturbances, although if hallucinations occur without intact reality testing, cannabis-induced psychotic disorder with hallucinations should be diagnosed.

Cannabis-Induced Mental Disorders

Cannabis-induced mental disorders are diverse. Besides intoxication (with or without perceptual disturbances, defined as hallucinations despite the presence of intact reality testing or illusions in the absence of delirium) and intoxication delirium, DSM-IV-TR specifically includes cannabis-induced psychotic disorder (with or without delusions) and cannabis-induced anxiety disorder. Cannabis-induced psychotic disorder with delusions is a syndrome (usually with persecutory delusions) that develops shortly after cannabis use. It may be associated with marked anxiety, depersonalization, and emotional lability and may be misdiagnosed as schizophrenia. Subsequent amnesia for the episode can occur. Acute adverse reactions to cannabis should be differentiated from symptoms of panic, major depressive episode, delusional disorder, bipolar disorder, or paranoid-type schizophrenia. Chronic use can also lead to symptoms resembling dysthymic disorder; individuals with a diagnosis of cannabis abuse are more likely to develop depressive symptoms than are those without a cannabis abuse diagnosis (Bovasso 2001).

Nicotine

Nicotine has euphoric effects and reinforcement properties similar to those of cocaine and opioids. Its effects can follow use of all forms of tobacco as well as use of medications containing nicotine (e.g., nicotine gum and patch). DSM-IV-TR includes no nicotine abuse or intoxication categories. It is notable that 25% of the population are smokers; 50%–80% of current smokers have nicotine dependence; and 50% of those who quit on their own experience withdrawal when they stop smoking (American Psychiatric Association 2000).

Nicotine Use Disorder

Nicotine Dependence

For nicotine, some of the generic criteria for substance dependence do not appear to apply, and other criteria require explanation. Tolerance is the absence of nausea, dizziness, and other characteristic symptoms despite the use of substantial amounts—or a diminished effect observed with continued use of the same amount—of the substance. In making the diagnosis, it should be recalled that spending a great deal of time attempting to procure nicotine is likely rare; however, excessive time spent actively smoking is exemplified by chain-smoking. An example of giving up important social, occupational, or recreational activities is the avoidance of an activity because it occurs in a smoking-restricted area.

Nicotine-Induced Disorder

Nicotine Withdrawal

Nicotine withdrawal is a characteristic syndrome that develops after abrupt cessation of, or reduction in, the use of nicotine, following a prolonged period (at least several weeks) of daily use. The withdrawal syndrome includes four or more of the following symptoms: dysphoric or depressed mood; insomnia; irritability, frustration, or anger; anxiety; difficulty concentrating; restlessness or impatience; decreased heart rate; and increased appetite (especially for sweets) or weight gain. Heart rate decreases by 5–12 beats per minute in the first few days after cessation, and weight increases an average of 2–3 kg in the year after cessation. Mild withdrawal may occur after switching to low-tar/low-nicotine cigarettes or after stopping the use of chewing tobacco, nicotine gum, or patches. Symptoms usually last 3–4 weeks, although the symptoms of craving may last approximately 6 months. During nicotine withdrawal, EEG changes may be seen, as well as alterations in rapid eye movement sleep and reductions in metabolic rate.

Differential Diagnosis of Nicotine Withdrawal

The symptoms of nicotine withdrawal overlap with those of other withdrawal syndromes as well as with symptoms of caffeine intoxication; anxiety, mood, and sleep disorders; and medication-induced akathisia. Reduction of symptoms on replacement of nicotine confirms the diagnosis.

Inhalants

The class of inhaled substances includes the aliphatic and aromatic hydrocarbons found in substances such as gasoline, glue, paint thinners, and spray paints. Less commonly used are halogenated hydrocarbons (in cleaners, correction fluid, spray-can propellants) and other volatile compounds containing esters, ketones, and glycols. It is usually difficult to determine the exact substance responsible for the disorder. Diagnosis is always confirmed by toxicology. Although there may be subtle differences in the effects of the compounds, not enough is known about their effects to distinguish among them. Indeed these drugs may be used interchangeably, and use may depend on availability and experience. Nonetheless, all are capable of producing dependence, abuse, and intoxication. There are no specific criteria sets for dependence or abuse of inhalants. This is partially the result of the uncertain existence of tolerance or withdrawal syndromes. A possible withdrawal syndrome beginning 24–48 hours after cessation of use and lasting 2–5 days has been described, with symptoms including sleep disturbances, tremor, irritability, diaphoresis, nausea, and fleeting illusions.

Inhalant-Induced Disorders

Inhalant Intoxication

Inhalant intoxication is clinically significant maladaptive behavioral or psychological changes (e.g., belligerence, assaultiveness, apathy, impaired judgment, impaired social or occupational functioning) that develop during or shortly after exposure. The maladaptive changes are accompanied by signs that include dizziness or visual disturbances (blurred vision or diplopia), nystagmus, incoordination, slurred speech, unsteady gait, tremor, and euphoria. Higher doses of inhalants may lead to the development of lethargy and psychomotor retardation, generalized muscle weakness, depressed reflexes, stupor, or coma.

Differential Diagnosis of Inhalant-Induced Disorders

Inhalant-induced disorders may be characterized by symptoms that resemble primary mental disorders. Mild to moderate intoxication can be similar to intoxication from alcohol, sedatives, hypnotics, or anxiolytics. Chronic users are likely to use other substances frequently and heavily, further complicating the diagnosis. History of the drug used and characteristic findings (including odor of solvent or paint residue) may differentiate inhalant intoxication from other substance intoxications. Rapid onset and resolution may also differentiate inhalant intoxication from other mental disorders and neurological conditions. Industrial workers may occasionally be accidentally exposed to volatile chemicals and suffer physiological intoxication. For such toxin exposures, the appropriate category is *other substance-related disorders.*

Caffeine

Caffeine is widely used in the form of coffee, tea, cola, chocolate, and cocoa and is also present in over-the-counter analgesics, cold preparations, and stimulants. There are no DSM-IV-TR diagnostic criteria for caffeine dependence or abuse. Withdrawal headaches may occur, but they are usually not severe enough to require treatment.

Caffeine-Induced Disorders

Caffeine Intoxication

Intoxication can lead to restlessness, nervousness, excitement, insomnia, flushing, diuresis, and gastrointestinal complaints. Doses leading to intoxication can vary. At high doses, there can be psychosis, arrhythmias, and psychomotor agitation. Mild sensory disturbances can occur at higher doses; at enormous doses, grand mal seizures and respiratory failure may occur. Because of tolerance, intoxication may not occur despite high caffeine intake.

Other Caffeine-Induced Disorders

DSM-IV-TR–recognized "other caffeine-induced disorders" include caffeine-induced anxiety disorder and caffeine-induced sleep disorder; a category for caffeine-related disorder not otherwise specified is also provided. In addition, DSM-IV-TR includes criteria for caffeine withdrawal.

Differential Diagnosis of Caffeine-Induced Disorders

The bulk of disorders requiring differentiation from caffeine-induced mental disorders are medical conditions that mimic caffeine intoxication. The temporal relationship of the symptoms to increased caffeine use or to abstinence from caffeine helps to establish the diagnosis. Manic episodes; panic disorder;

generalized anxiety disorder; amphetamine intoxication; sedative, hypnotic, or anxiolytic withdrawal or nicotine withdrawal; sleep disorders; and medication-induced side effects (e.g., akathisia) can cause a clinical picture that is similar to that of caffeine intoxication.

Other (or Unknown) Substance–Related Disorders

DSM-IV-TR includes categories for dependence, abuse, intoxication, withdrawal, delirium, psychosis with delusions, psychosis with hallucinations, alcohol-induced persisting dementia or amnesia, disordered mood, anxiety, sexual dysfunction, and disordered sleep that result from use of substances such as amyl nitrate, anticholinergics, gamma-hydroxybutyrate (GHB), corticosteroids, anabolic steroids, antihistamines, and antiparkinsonian agents, as well as substances whose identity is unknown at the time of patient presentation.

GHB is a CNS depressant used in some countries (but not the United States) as an anesthetic. It is increasingly used worldwide as a recreational drug by party and nightclub attendees and bodybuilders, and it also may be used as a "date rape" drug. It has been marketed to bodybuilders as a growth hormone releaser. Known as "liquid ecstasy" or "cherry meth," GHB increases CNS dopamine levels and has effects on the endogenous opioid system. GHB toxicity manifests as coma, seizures, respiratory depression, vomiting, anesthesia, and amnesia (Drasbek et al. 2006). Although full recovery usually occurs, the toxic state can be life-threatening.

Polysubstance Dependence

Polysubstance dependence is the DSM-IV-TR category diagnosed when an individual has over the past year repeatedly used substances from at least three classes (with the exception of nicotine and caffeine) without one predominating. Dependence is global—not for any one drug. Patients often downplay use of these secondary drugs. For example, a diagnosed cocaine abuser may suddenly develop alcohol withdrawal. Without a thorough substance use history, onset of these unexpected symptoms can take the treatment team by surprise.

Drug Combinations

Often one drug is used in combination to counterbalance the side effects or to potentiate the effect of another drug. "Speedballing," the intravenous combination of heroin and cocaine, is lethal but is known to mute cocaine dysphoria. Glutethimide (Doriden) and cocaine are often combined, potentiating respiratory depression. Pentazocine (Talwin) and diphenhydramine (Benadryl)—together called "T's and blues"—are prescription medications that produce intoxication when combined. Virtually any combination of alcohol and other drugs may be seen. Marijuana use is often so pervasive among polysubstance abusers that it is not even perceived as a drug of abuse.

Establishing a Diagnosis: Dilemmas, Signs, and Countertransference

Diagnostic Dilemmas

The substance-abusing patient presents with medical, neurological, and psychiatric disturbances that need careful systematic assessment. The challenges of differential diagnosis should instill some degree of humility and conservatism in the clinician. Conservative management with a careful review of medical, psychiatric, and substance abuse histories; physical and mental status examinations; laboratory tests; and third-party information can clarify the diagnosis. In other cases, only time and observation can clarify the etiology.

Signs and Symptoms

Accurate diagnosis and appropriate care for substance-abusing patients require attention to physical signs and symptoms. At the outset, when differentiating among overdose, withdrawal, chronic organicity, or psychiatric diagnoses, one should rule out or treat life-threatening conditions first. For example, tachycardia and fever may indicate infection, withdrawal, or drug toxicity. An abnormal pulse may indicate intoxication with sympathomimetic drugs, withdrawal from CNS depressants, or arrhythmia from overdose. Bradycardia could indicate opioid intoxication, severe head trauma, or cardiac conduction delays. Abnormal pupil size or oculogyric movements can help clarify various drug overdose situations. Pinpoint pupils in a comatose patient may signal opioid overdose. Mydriasis is associated with sympathomimetic intoxication. Gaze palsies, confusion, and ataxia could be due to thiamine deficiency leading to Wernicke's encephalopathy. Nystagmus occurs in PCP intoxication. Physical examination can detect fresh needle marks, recent alcohol intake, or nasal irritation from cocaine or inhalant abuse. Of course, substance-abusing patients frequently have comorbid medical and neurological conditions that affect mental and physical status, such as acquired immunodeficiency syndrome (AIDS) dementia, seizures, head trauma, and infections, and these conditions should be considered.

Markedly altered mental status, evidence of recent substance intake, and reliable corroborating history can aid in distinguishing among withdrawal, chronic organicity, and functional diagnoses. Diagnosis may be delayed or provisional in patients with a known chronic substance abuse history, unreliable recent history, and history of major psychiatric symptoms. Undocumented organicity can confound diagnosis. Alcohol dementia and postconcussive head syndromes can sensitize the brain to react to minor substance abuse with dramatic and unpredictable results. In such patients, many things are ongoing concurrently. It is important to provide a safe environment, to protect the patient and others from harm, and to ensure basic airway, respiratory, and cardiac support until a general diagnostic workup is completed.

Countertransference and Diagnosis

SUD patients with histrionic, paranoid, borderline, or antisocial features may present with an exacerbation of primitive defenses (e.g., projection, projective identification, splitting) during intoxication. These patients may be belligerent, distrustful, unappreciative, uncooperative, or violent, making management and history-taking difficult. Due to the strong countertransference such patients evoke, inappropriate diagnostic and treatment decisions may ensue. Before making an unusual treatment decision or participating in uncharacteristic behavior with a patient, it may be helpful for the therapist to consult with another expert, and sometimes a team approach is especially useful. A simple "time-out" for the therapist to collect his or her thoughts and feelings may be helpful. Countertransference feelings should not be ignored; rather, they should be used to help clarify the diagnosis. Frequently, a patient's obnoxious, uncooperative, destructive behavior or apparent personality problems are time-limited and related to the substance-induced state. They may reflect the patient's fear and low self-esteem. A totally uncooperative patient, if tolerated through acute intoxication, can have a dramatic and unexpected turnaround.

Psychiatric Comorbidity

"Dual diagnosis" ("co-occurring state") patients have an SUD and another major psychiatric diagnosis. The connections between the two may be manifold (Mueser et al. 1998). Major psychiatric disorders may precede the development of substance abuse, develop concurrently, or manifest secondarily. Psychiatric disorders may precipitate the onset or modify the course of an SUD. Psychiatric disorders and substance abuse may present as independent conditions. Thus, it is difficult at any one point in time to differentiate symptoms of withdrawal, intoxication, and secondary cognitive, affective, perceptual, or personality changes from underlying psychiatric disorders. Important tools in differential diagnosis include careful history-taking, urine screens, and determination of the course or sequence of symptoms. Information obtained from third parties, including family history, is critical.

Substance Abuse and Affective Disorders

Regardless of the patient's earlier experiences of euphoria during substance use, chronic major depression occurs late in the course of addiction. This may be the result of altered neurochemistry, hormonal or metabolic changes, chronic demoralization, grief from personal losses, or the stresses of the addictive lifestyle. Chronic heroin use often leads to lethargy and social withdrawal. Sustained alcohol use generally produces depression and anxiety, although brief periods of euphoria may still occur.

It is vital to differentiate between alcohol-induced depressive disorder and primary depressive disorder. According to one large study, subjects with primary major depressive episodes were more likely to be female, white, and married; to have had experience with fewer drugs and less treatment for alcoholism; to have attempted suicide; and to have a close relative with a major mood disorder (Schuckit et al. 1997). Although the majority of alcoholics will not have an independent diagnosis of major depressive disorder, other less severe depressive disorders may persist in a large proportion of alcoholics after cessation of drinking. Drinking may be more of a problem during the hypomanic or manic phase of bipolar disorder than during the depressed phase. In the majority of cases, depressive symptomatology subsides after 3–4 weeks of abstinence and usually needs no pharmacological intervention. Use of antidepressants is indicated after a drug-free period, and abstinence is required for efficacy. Untreated major depression in a primary alcoholic or secondary alcoholism in a primary depressive patient worsens prognosis.

There is considerable evidence that depression has a higher incidence in active opioid users and may subside with abstinence. The prevalence of major depression ranges from 17% to 30% among heroin addicts and is considerably higher among methadone clients. Estimates of the prevalence of affective disorders among substance-using patients in general have ranged as high as 60%. Many depressive episodes are mild and related to stress; they may be associated with treatment seeking. In a 2½-year follow-up study, depression was found to be a poor prognostic sign, except in cases of coexisting antisocial personality disorder, in which the presence of depression improved prognosis (Brooner et al. 1997).

Concurrent affective disorders have been reported in 30% of cocaine addicts, with a significant proportion of these patients having bipolar disorder or cyclothymia. Bipolar patients in a manic phase may use cocaine to heighten feelings of grandiosity. The profound dysphoric mood related to cocaine binges will resolve in the majority of cocaine addicts. A minority of patients may have underlying unipolar or bipolar disorder, which needs to be treated separately. This abstinence dysphoria may be secondary to depletion of brain catecholamines (e.g., dopamine) or to alteration in neural receptors, with resultant postsynaptic supersensitivity. Some authors have suggested that comorbid cocaine abuse may be a robust predictor of poor outcome among depressed alcoholics. Concurrent major depressive disorder reduces the risk of successful remission from substance dependence and predicts relapse. As a result, ongoing attention to both conditions is important, even if their medication treatment is sequential (Hasin et al. 2002). An armamentarium of coping skills, a greater number of positive life events, and family support are positive prognostic factors (Brooner et al. 1997).

Substance Abuse and Psychosis

Psychotic symptomatology can result from the use of a wide range of psychoactive substances: alcohol, cocaine, PCP, hallucinogens, and inhalants. As noted previously, all abused substances have "organic" syndromes that mimic various functional psychiatric syndromes. Opioids, however, have shown some antipsychotic properties.

More complex is the relationship between schizophrenia and substance abuse. Various studies have shown that 50%–60% of patients with schizophrenia and 60%–80% of those with bipolar disorder abuse substances (Schneier and Siris 1987). The role of substance abuse in precipitating or altering the course of an underlying schizophrenic disorder is unclear. Substance abuse may exacerbate symptoms in well-controlled schizophrenics. Alcohol, marijuana, hallucinogen, or cocaine abuse may produce psychotic symptoms that persist only in vulnerable individuals. It may be that patients with schizophrenia seek out certain types of drugs for self-medication and for self-treatment of medication side effects. Persons with schizophrenia also use tobacco and caffeine more often than do control populations. Tobacco use has been associated with lowering of blood levels of antipsychotics and leads to a need for higher-than-average doses of antipsychotics for symptom control. Schizophrenia patients may seek out drugs that increase the chance of precipitating psychotic episodes to feel a sense of mastery or to experience merging. Schizophrenia patients may be treating dysphoria, or negative symptoms of their disease, and use stimulants to allow them to feel more intensely. These patients may also be treating extrapyramidal or sedative side effects of antipsychotic medications. Schizophrenia patients who abuse stimulant drugs may also be treating an independent, underlying affective disorder. Substance abuse may provide the schizophrenia patient with the experience of control over unpredictable states of consciousness or may provide a strong identity as a substance abuser, which may be more palatable and perceived as being less stigmatic than having a major psychiatric disorder. Conversely, a lower degree of ego strength may contribute to greater experiences of craving and lesser capacities to resist cocaine, and probably other substances, among persons with schizophrenia (Schneier and Siris 1987).

Substance Abuse and Anxiety Disorders

Generalized anxiety disorder, posttraumatic stress disorder (PTSD), panic disorder, and phobic disorder are overrepresented in substance abuse patients, especially alcoholics and sedative-hypnotic abusers. A study in alcoholic patients reported generalized anxiety disorder in 9% and phobias in 3%, rates significantly higher than in the general population (Ross et al. 1988). PTSD has been related to the high rates of alcoholism in Vietnam veterans who saw active duty. Panic disorder has been found in 5% of inpatient addicts (Compton et al. 2007). Benzodiazepine doses of up to 1,000–1,500 mg have been reported in patients with underlying anxiety disorders. These patients are often very difficult to treat because of the complex interaction between the anxiety disorder and the SUD. In treatment of addicted patients with anxiety disorders, benzodiazepines should be avoided if possible. Specific treatment of the underlying anxiety disorder may include typical and low-dose atypical antipsychotics, antidepressants, monoamine oxidase inhibitors, buspirone, gabapentin, or propranolol (see Chapter 12, "Treatment Modalities").

Although many patients with preexisting anxiety disorders experience alcohol use as self-medication, alcohol use can in fact exacerbate an underlying anxiety disorder and alter its course. Self-medication with abusable substances often occurs during war and disaster (Greiger et al. 2003).

Substance Abuse and Eating Disorders

The clinician should be aware of the high rate of alcohol use among individuals with eating disorders; this relationship is likely related to the anxiety experienced by the perfectionistic, impulsive, or dramatic traits seen in this group. Usually, the eating disorder develops first; use is more common in those with bulimic type of anorexia nervosa, or in bulimia itself, than in anorexia itself (Bulik et al. 2004). Given the possibility of malnutrition-induced metabolic or hematological derangements, use of laboratory studies in this population requires great caution and attention.

Substance Abuse and Neuropsychiatric Impairment

Chronic abuse of alcohol, sedatives, and inhalants has been well correlated with chronic brain damage and neuropsychological impairment. These impairments may be gross, as evidenced in alcohol dementia or Korsakoff's syndrome, or relatively mild and detected only by neuropsychological testing. Cognitive impairment may be short-lived and may recede after 3–4 weeks of abstinence, improve gradually over several months or years of abstinence, or be permanent. Alcohol's damage to brain tissue has been chronicled by abnormal computed tomography scan findings (cortical atrophy, which may reverse as well), EEG changes (decreased alpha activity), and alterations in auditory evoked potentials (decreased P300 amplitude). In the case of benzodiazepine abuse, however, the cognitive impairment may be reversible (Salzman et al. 1992).

Key Points

- Diagnoses in substance-related conditions can be very specific according to substance.
- DSM prompts recognition of multiple comorbid conditions that should be diagnosed when appropriate.
- DSM prompts concurrent diagnoses related to a particular substance and describes which should be considered.
- Identification of specific substance-induced states can be lifesaving.

References

American Psychiatric Association: Diagnostic and Statistical Manual of Mental Disorders, 3rd Edition. Washington, DC, American Psychiatric Association, 1980

American Psychiatric Association: Diagnostic and Statistical Manual of Mental Disorders, 4th Edition. Washington, DC, American Psychiatric Association, 1994

American Psychiatric Association: Diagnostic and Statistical Manual of Mental Disorders, 4th Edition, Text Revision. Washington, DC, American Psychiatric Association, 2000

Bovasso GB: Cannabis abuse as a risk factor for depressive symptoms. Am J Psychiatry 158:2033–2037, 2001

Brooner RK, King VL, Kidorf M, et al: Psychiatric and substance use comorbidity among treatment seeking opioid abusers. Arch Gen Psychiatry 54:71–80, 1997

Budney AJ, Hughes JR: The cannabis withdrawal syndrome. Curr Opin Psychiatry 19:233–238, 2006

Bulik CM, Klump CL, Thornton L, et al: Alcohol use disorder comorbidity in eating disorders: a multicenter study. J Clin Psychiatry 65:1000–1006, 2004

Caton CLM, Drake RE, Hasin DS, et al: Differences between early-phase primary psychotic disorders with concurrent substance use and substance-induced psychoses. Arch Gen Psychiatry 62:137–145, 2005

Compton WM, Thomas YF, Stinson FS, et al: Prevalence, correlates, disability, and comorbidity of DSM-IV drug abuse and dependence in the United States: results from the National Epidemiologic Survey on Alcohol and Related Conditions. Arch Gen Psychiatry 64:566–576, 2007

De Bruijn C, Van den Brink W, de Graaf R, et al: Alcohol abuse and dependence criteria as predictors of a chronic course of alcohol use disorders in the general population. Alcohol Alcohol 40:441–446, 2005

Drasbek KR, Christensen J, Jensen K: Gamma-hydroxybutyrate—a drug of abuse. Acta Neurol Scand 114:145–156, 2006

Greiger TA, Fullerton CS, Ursano RJ: Posttraumatic stress disorder, alcohol use, and perceived safety after the terrorist attack on the Pentagon. Psychiatr Serv 54:1380–1382, 2003

Hasin D, Liu X, Nunes E, et al: Effects of major depression on remission and relapse of substance dependence. Arch Gen Psychiatry 59:375–380, 2002

Mueser KT, Drake RD, Wallach MA: Dual diagnosis: a review of etiological theories. Addict Behav 23:717–734, 1998

Ross HE, Glaser FB, Germanson T: The prevalence of psychiatric disorders in patients with alcohol and other drug problems. Arch Gen Psychiatry 45:1023–1031, 1988

Salzman C, Fisher J, Nobel K, et al: Cognitive improvement following benzodiazepine discontinuation in elderly nursing home residents. Int J Geriatr Psychiatry 7:89–93, 1992

Schneier FR, Siris SG: A review of psychoactive substance use and abuse in schizophrenia: patterns of drug choice. J Nerv Ment Dis 175:641–652, 1987

Schnoll SH: Cocaine and stimulants, in Clinical Textbook of Addictive Disorders, 3rd Edition. Edited by Frances RJ, Mack AH, Miller SI. New York, Guilford, 2005, pp 184–218

Schuckit MA, Tipp JE, Bergman M, et al: Comparison of induced and independent major depressive disorders in 2,945 alcoholics. Am J Psychiatry 154:948–957, 1997

Spitzer RL, Williams JBW, Gibbon M: Structured Clinical Interview for DSM-IV. New York, New York State Psychiatric Institute, Biometrics Research, 1995

6

Natural Histories
of Substance Abuse

Alcohol

The signs and symptoms of alcoholism can be strikingly consistent among individuals in the late stages of the disease. However, with the concept of "case heterogeneity" in mind, there appear to be subtypes of alcoholism characterized by differences in age at onset, underlying etiology, degree of hereditary influence, social and cultural background, and natural outcome. Vaillant (1996) conducted one of the few prospective longitudinal studies of alcoholic individuals. In his studies, many alcoholics continued to drink until death, some stopped drinking, and others showed a pattern of long abstinence followed by relapses. This pattern holds true not just for those who are dependent on alcohol but also for those who demonstrate other types of problem use, such as binge drinking, which, like alcohol dependence, can progress from adolescence to adulthood (McCarty et al. 2004).

Although it is true that alcoholism is often a progressive disease that may continue without remission throughout the course of someone's life, some medical personnel have an unduly pessimistic view of the natural course of alcoholism and believe that an alcoholic will never get better, even with treatment. At the other extreme, some family members have an unrealistically hopeful view and believe that the alcoholic will stop drinking in the near future without help. Large-scale outcome studies suggest that approximately 30% of alcoholics will, at some point in the course of their illness, achieve stable abstinence without any form of treatment (Armor et al. 1978). This percentage improves in some studies to approximately 70% with some form of treatment. Treatment may include professional treatment and/or self-help groups. Vaillant (1996) also described a series of natural healing forces (e.g., church involvement, fear of medical complications, fear of family loss) that may substitute for some aspects of formal treatment through the meeting of dependency needs. Vaillant found that 5 years of abstinence from alcohol predicted long-term success and that chances of relapse at that point are similar to the chances of developing a problem in the general population.

Thus, it is important to understand alcoholism as a disease that has many different patterns and is characterized by relapses. Examples include an elderly woman who begins drinking habitually after the death of her husband; a surgeon who drinks pathologically for a period of time, but when faced with the loss of her practice, receives treatment and recovers; and an individual with a job and family who loses everything due to drinking, becomes homeless for several years, but eventually, through involvement with Alcoholics Anonymous (AA), regains his job and family. Some alcoholics never develop serious medical problems; the majority never seek treatment.

Classifying Alcoholism

There are important aspects of alcohol use disorders that should be analyzed. Jellinek (1960) was the first to describe subgroups of alcoholics, distinguishing between individuals who engaged in persistent alcohol-seeking behaviors and individuals who could abstain from alcohol for long periods of time but quickly lost control and could not terminate intake after resumption of drinking. Cloninger et al. (1996) described two subtypes of alcoholics. Type I alcoholic individuals generally start intake with heavy drinking reinforced by external circumstances after the age of 25 years; have greater ability to abstain for long periods of time; and frequently feel loss of control, guilt, and fear about their alcohol dependency. Type II alcoholic individuals generally have an early onset (before the age of 25 years) of problem drinking and show spontaneous alcohol-seeking behavior regardless of their external circumstances. They have conduct problems and only infrequently experience feelings of loss of control, guilt, or fear in regard to their alcohol dependency. Interestingly, research on the efficacy of the drug ondansetron in preventing relapse revealed differences in response between these two groups. An early age at onset of drinking behavior is associated with a rate of lifetime alcohol dependence that is significantly higher than in those who start drinking after the age of 21 years (Hingson et al. 2006).

Newer findings on the relationship between alcohol abuse and dependence have shown some surprising and valuable results. Cohort studies on long-term alcohol use do not support that alcohol abuse is a precursor to alcohol dependence. In one study in which use was observed over 5 years in 300 subjects, only 3.5% of the patients who had met criteria for abuse at the baseline assessment met criteria for dependence after 5 years. As a comparison, 2.5% of control subjects who had no evidence of an alcohol use disorder at baseline met criteria for alcohol dependence after 5 years (Schuckit et al. 2001).

Medical Complications

Adverse physical effects of chronic alcohol abuse include organic mental disorders, diseases of the digestive tract (including liver disease, gastritis, ulcer, pancreatitis, and gastrointestinal cancers), bone marrow suppression, and muscle and hormone changes. Alcohol has direct toxic effects on the brain, which, combined with metabolic, traumatic, and nutritional deficits, may cause various alcohol-related mental disorders (discussed in Chapter 5, "Definition, Presentation, and Diagnosis"). Alcohol intake can cause progressive liver damage. Fatty liver develops in nearly anyone with sufficient alcohol intake. Serious alcoholic hepatitis, which can have a 5-year mortality rate of up to 50%, may develop. Liver cirrhosis occurs in only about 10% of alcoholics; however, 11,000 die from liver disease annually. Of patients with chronic pancreatitis, 75% have an alcohol use disorder. Alcohol dissolves mucus and irritates the gastric lining, which contributes to bleeding. Every alcoholic should have a rectal exam with a stool guaiac test as part of a complete physical exam (Lieber 1995).

Alcohol use, heavy tobacco use, and deficiencies of vitamins A and B all contribute to high rates of cancer of the mouth, tongue, larynx, esophagus, stomach, liver, and pancreas. Alcoholic patients with oral cancer (to which alcohol significantly contributes) tend to delay seeking treatment longer than most other cancer patients. Early detection is particularly crucial in these diseases. Alcoholic cardiomyopathy can develop after 10 or more years of drinking. Abstinence contributes to recovery in those cases in which damage is not too extensive. Alcohol also has chronic effects on other muscle tissue.

Effects on Blood

Alcoholism is part of the differential diagnosis for anemia, especially megaloblastic anemia. Because of reduced white cell count or further damage to immune functioning, the effects of continued heavy drinking on the possible progression and susceptibility to infection by human immunodeficiency virus (HIV) and progression to acquired immunodeficiency syndrome (AIDS) are being studied. For similar reasons, other infectious diseases (e.g., tuberculosis, bacterial pneumonia) have been common among those with alcoholism.

Effects on Hormones

Alcohol interferes with male sexual function and fertility directly through effects on testosterone levels and indirectly through testicular atrophy. Relatively increased levels of estrogen lead to development of gynecomastia and body hair loss. Sexual functioning is affected indirectly through the impact of alcohol on the limbic system and the hypothalamic-pituitary axis. This may be due to vitamin B deficiency or direct toxic effects of alcohol. In women there also may be severe gonadal failure, with an inability to produce adequate quantities of female hormones, affecting secondary sexual characteristics, reducing menstruation, and producing infertility.

Additional Complications

Alcoholism tends to increase blood pressure and is associated with increased risk of cerebrovascular accidents. Alcoholic cerebellar degeneration is a slowly evolving condition encountered along with long-standing histories of excessive use. It affects the cerebellar cortex and produces truncal ataxia and gait disturbances. Alcoholic peripheral neuropathy is characterized by a stocking-and-glove paresthesia, with decreased reflexes and autonomic nerve dysfunction causing, among other problems, impotence. Central pontine myelinolysis is a rare neurological condition of unknown etiology and high mortality. Also of unknown etiology, Marchiafava-Bignami disease is a rare demyelinating disease of the corpus callosum. Computed tomography (CT) studies have shown that the brain changes resulting from alcohol use may be reversible in as little as 3 weeks (Crews et al. 2005). Alcohol may also impair parasympathetic nerve functioning, which may affect the ability to maintain an erection.

Risks of Alcohol Withdrawal

Besides seizures, delirium tremens, and stroke, various medical complications may ensue from being in alcohol withdrawal, such as cardiomyopathy, pancreatitis, hypoglycemia, gastrointestinal bleeding, hepatic failure, and encephalopathy.

Possible Benefits of Moderate Alcohol Use

Although data have shown that moderate alcohol intake may benefit various medical conditions, such as ischemic myocardial infarction or stroke, discussions with patients should include mindfulness of the various medical complications of alcohol and the dangers of excessive use.

Sedatives, Hypnotics, and Anxiolytics

The course of central nervous system (CNS) depressant abuse/dependence varies from long prodromal periods of use with benzodiazepines or hypnotics, to more rapid onset of addiction with barbiturates, or episodic abuse with other CNS depressants such as methaqualone (Quaalude) or ethchlorvynol (Placidyl). Combinations of CNS depressants with alcohol or opioids can potentiate the level of intoxication, respiratory depression, and mortality. Chronic sedative abuse can produce blackouts and neuropsychological damage similar to that seen in alcoholism (Caplan et al. 2007). Patients who began using sedatives to treat anxiety will experience an initial anxiety rebound on discontinuation of these agents, which in most patients is similar to withdrawal in terms of course and symptomatology.

Opioids

Intoxication and Withdrawal

Intravenous heroin or opioid intoxication produces a subjective euphoric rush that can be highly reinforcing. Opioid users describe this rush as a feeling of warmth or as an oceanic feeling. The daily use of opioids over days to weeks, depending on the dose and potency of the drug, will produce opioid withdrawal symptoms on cessation of use.

Neonatal Opioid Withdrawal

A syndrome of narcotic abstinence is reported in up to 90% of neonates of mothers addicted to opioids (American Academy of Pediatrics Committee on Drugs 1998). Although the baby may appear normal at or shortly after birth, symptoms may appear 12–24 hours later, depending on the half-life of the opioid, and may persist for several months. The full-blown syndrome can include hyperactivity, tremors, seizures, hyperactive reflexes, gastrointestinal dysfunction, respiratory dysfunction, and vague autonomic symptoms (e.g., yawning, sneezing, sweating, nasal congestion, increased lacrimation, fever). Long-term residual symptoms include infants appearing anxious, hard to please, hyperactive, and emotionally labile.

Adverse Physical Effects

Contaminated needles and impure drugs can lead to endocarditis, septicemia, pulmonary emboli, and pulmonary hypertension. Contaminants can cause skin infections, hepatitis B, and spread of HIV. Death rates in young addicts are increased 20-fold by infection, homicide, suicide, overdose, and (recently) AIDS. Opioid overdose should be suspected in any undiagnosed coma patient, especially along with respiratory depression, pupillary constriction, or presence of needle marks.

Basic research advances in identification of distinct subtypes of opioid receptors have provided increased understanding of the mechanism of cellular opioid neuroregulation and physiology. Cellular mechanisms of opioid receptors are being explored in relation to characteristics of opioid receptors and intracellular modulators of opioid action. Multiple subtypes of opioid receptors designated as *mu, delta, kappa, sigma,* and *epsilon* have been described.

Neuroadaptation at receptor sites has been hypothesized to produce tolerance and dependence.

Psychosocial Features of Opioid Use

Kandel and Faust (1975) studied patterns of psychoactive substance abuse extensively in adolescents and young adults and found a progression from tobacco, alcohol, and marijuana to sedatives, cocaine, and opioids. Regular marijuana use, development of depressive symptoms, lack of closeness to parents, and dropping out of school may predispose an individual to later narcotic use. Often, opioid abuse is endemic to economically disadvantaged communities that have high rates of unemployment, low levels of family stability, and increased tolerance of criminality. These social stressors may result in hopelessness, low self-esteem, poor self-concept, and identification with drug-involved role models and may be intervening variables in the increased opioid dependency rates in minorities. Where poverty and high rates of unemployment are prevalent, many individuals may feel they have little to lose in experimenting with drugs, and conventional scare tactics have little impact. Alienation from social institutions such as school, increased social deviancy, and impulsivity are high-risk characteristics. There exists a clear association between heroin use and crime. The overwhelming majority of inner-city community members, however, are not opioid users. Research examining factors protective for individuals at risk is important.

The Self-Medication Hypothesis

In research initially centered on opioid users, Khantzian (1997) observed a strong interaction between dominant dysphoric feelings and drug preference. Recent updates to this hypothesis suggest that although self-medication partially explains the initiation and continuation of substance abuse, a wider array of factors are actually at work (Henwood and Padgett 2007). The self-medication hypothesis posits that the individual self-selects drugs on the basis of personality and ego impairments. For example, Khantzian emphasized an "antirage property of opioids" that provides a pharmacological solution or defense against overwhelming anger because of either deficient ego defenses or low frustration tolerance. Patients may self-medicate to alleviate symptoms of anxiety, depression, or attention-deficit/hyperactivity disorder (ADHD) or to counteract antipsychotic medication side effects or the effects of other medications, and they may use specific drugs to achieve specific effects. Patients may seek mastery over pain through self-administered drug titration of withdrawal and dysphoria. Even in the absence of a diagnosable psychiatric disorder, it is plausible that substances serve as "medication" for unwanted symptoms. Naltrexone has reduced alcohol use in those who experienced increased use during periods of both mood elevation and depression (Kranzler et al. 2004).

Progression of Addiction

The course of heroin addiction generally involves a 2- to 6-year interval between regular heroin use and seeking of treatment. Early experimentation with opioids may not lead to opioid addiction, but once addiction develops, a lifelong pattern of use and relapse frequently ensues. A preexisting personality disorder may be a factor for drug use progression. The need to secure the drug predisposes the addict to participate in illegal activities or complicates an already existing tendency toward criminality.

Cocaine

Natural Course

The majority of casual (especially intranasal) cocaine users do not become dependent, but the widespread thinking in the late 1970s that cocaine was not addictive was mistaken. It is only recently that researchers have begun to look at different characteristics associated with an increased likelihood that the user will progress from abuse to dependence. For example, one recent study revealed that men were more likely than women to relapse after a period of abstinence (Gallop et al. 2007). The time period from first use to addiction is usually about 4 years with intranasal use in adults; however, it may be as little as 1½ years in adolescents. With availability of more potent cocaine derivatives (e.g., crack cocaine), experimentation may result in presentation for treatment within months. Most cocaine addicts describe the initial experimentation with cocaine as having been fun. At some point in the experience, cocaine use is no longer fun, but joyless and compulsive. The activating properties of the drug become more prominent as the euphoria wanes. Consumption of cocaine, initially done in public places such as in bars and at parties, may become an isolating, alienating experience associated with considerable paranoia. Data from the Centers for Disease Control and Prevention's National Violent Death Reporting System indicated that in 2005, 7.6% of suicide completers who were screened for cocaine tested positive (Karch et al. 2008).

Chronic Use

Chronic cocaine use depletes all neurotransmitters and leads to increased receptor sensitivity to dopamine and norepinephrine. These changes are associated with depression, fatigue, poor attention to self-care, poor self-esteem, poor libido, and mild parkinsonism. Tolerance to cocaine does occur, and with continued use, psychosis, an acquired ADHD-like syndrome, and/or stereotyped behaviors become apparent. Given the "fluffy" findings on positron emission tomography (PET) scans in such patients, it is assumed that this state is correlated with tissue pathology. Ongoing research in heavy cocaine users has focused on the drug's pathological effects on a variety of other processes, including myelination.

Because of the high cost of cocaine, financial and legal problems may be the first sign of trouble before other stigmas of dependence develop. A loss of control, exaggerated involvement, and continued use despite adverse social, occupational, and health effects are criteria pointing to a diagnosis of cocaine dependency.

Adverse Medical Effects

Cocaine has been associated with acute and chronic ailments. Chronic intranasal use has led to nasoseptal defects due to vasoconstriction. Vasodilation also produces nasal stuffiness or "the runs." There is evidence of long-term cerebrovascular disease secondary to chronic cocaine use (Nanda et al. 2006). Anesthetic properties of cocaine may lead to oral numbness and dental neglect. Malnutrition, severe weight loss, and dehydration often result from cocaine binges. Intravenous use of cocaine complicated by impurities may produce endocarditis, septicemia, HIV spread, local vasculitis, hepatitis B, emphysema, pulmonary emboli, and granulomas. Freebase cocaine has been associated with decreased pulmonary exchange, and pulmonary dysfunction may persist. Cocaine injection sites are characterized by prominent ecchymoses; opioid injection sites more frequently show needle marks.

Positive cocaine urine test results have been increasingly found in homicide victims, in individuals arrested for murder, and in persons who have died from overdose. Cocaine-induced fatalities have an average blood concentration of 6.2 mg/L (Spiehler and Reed 1985). Congenital deficiency of pseudocholinesterase may slow down the metabolism and result in toxic levels, sudden delirium, and hypothermia. Deaths in recreational low-dose users have been reported. Acute agitation, diaphoresis, tachycardia, metabolic and respiratory acidosis, cardiac arrhythmia, and grand mal seizures can lead ultimately to respiratory arrest. Recurrent myocardial infarction in cocaine use associated with tachycardia and coronary vasoconstriction has been reported. Subarachnoid hemorrhage may be precipitated in patients with underlying arterial venous malformations.

Pregnant women who use cocaine may have increased risks for placental abruption, and babies of mothers who use cocaine have been shown to have decreased interactive behavior on Brazelton scales. Further research is being done to study the teratogenicity of cocaine.

Amphetamines

Amphetamine abuse may start in conjunction with weight-loss treatment, attempts at energy enhancement, or more serious intravenous use. Amphetamine abuse by intravenous administration can present with the same medical complications as seen with intravenous cocaine or heroin use. Amphetamine use shares many signs, symptoms, and long-term sequelae with cocaine use. Stimulants such as methylphenidate (as well as cocaine) can induce enhancement of sexual desire, thereby increasing the probability of risky sexual activity (Volkow et al. 2007).

Methamphetamine, a synthetic stimulant drug that has risen in use starkly, is highly addictive and poses serious risks for users, including risks at the neurobiological level. Methamphetamine abuse is associated with various medical consequences, including HIV risk, and various psychiatric sequelae. Its effects stem from damage both to dopamine and serotonin systems. Damage to the dopamine system is long-lasting and is associated with some irreversible declines in neuropsychological function, particularly in terms of functions associated with the striatum, sometimes being expressed as amotivation or anhedonia (Wang et al. 2004). In addition, users tend to show increased levels of aggression, which has been seen as resulting from injury to serotonin metabolism (Sekine et al. 2006). By various mechanisms, methamphetamine may cause systemic or organ-specific damage, such as significant dental pathology, dermatological effects, cardiomegaly, microvascular disease, accelerated coronary artery disease, arrhythmias, myocardial infarction, and cardiomyopathy.

Phencyclidine

Chronic psychotic episodes are reported following use of phencyclidine (PCP). With the unpredictability of the experience, it is difficult to explain the manifestation of abuse of this substance in certain individuals. In contrast to the use of hallucinogens, use of PCP may lead to long-term neuropsychological deficits. PCP abuse may occur in conjunction with multiple substance abuse and may be associated with similar risk factors. Cases of pure PCP abuse have been reported, and in our experience these individuals appear to have significant psychopathology; however, it is difficult to distinguish drug effects from premorbid personality. PCP intoxication produces specific autonomic sequelae that are both sympathomimetic and cholinergic, as well as dysfunction of the cerebellar system, including horizontal nystagmus, ataxia, and dizziness.

Hallucinogens

Most hallucinogens can produce certain acute adverse effects. The "bad trip" is a syndrome of anxiety, panic, dysphoria, and paranoia that occurs during the period of intoxication. The fact that this syndrome can lead to suicidal ideation and attempts makes its identification important. There is no recognized withdrawal syndrome from hallucinogens. These drugs can also lead to chronic effects, including prolonged psychotic states that resemble psychosis or mania. However, syndromes that last longer than 4–6 weeks are generally thought to represent an underlying primary psychiatric disease rather than a psychotic state secondary to hallucinogen use. Flashbacks are another chronic sequela of hallucinogens. Hallucinogens have been noted to produce flashback experiences in 15%–30% of chronic users. Prevalence of flashbacks increases with the number of times the individual seeks medical attention, except during acute intoxication or disturbing flashbacks that may be precipitated by other substances, such as marijuana. Most strikingly, some hallucinogens have produced permanent parkinsonism in users through selective destruction of the substantia nigra. There is less and less doubt that 3,4-methylenedioxymethamphetamine (MDMA or "Ecstasy") permanently affects neuropsychological function, despite ongoing attempts to present the substance as innocuous.

Cannabis

Use of marijuana tends to begin in adolescence, and the earlier the use begins, the more serious the problems that ensue (see Chapter 9, "Children and Adolescents," for further discussion of initiation). The use of alcohol and cigarettes may be associated with marijuana abuse. Cannabis use has been described as a stepping stone to the use of other illegal drugs (i.e., the gateway hypothesis), both in the United States and in other Western cultures, and this has now been shown by comparisons of use in monozygotic versus dizygotic twin pairs (Lynskey et al. 2003). Cannabis is often used in combinations with other substances (e.g., cocaine). Although many young people experiment with cannabis, actual abuse patterns tend to be associated with introduction to drug subcultures among youth, low parental supervision, parental substance abuse, and abuse of drugs by peers. Cannabis abuse should be suspected in someone who has a characteristic set of symptoms, including loss of communication with family, erratic mood changes, deterioration of moral values, apathy, change in friends, truancy, academic underachievement, denial of use even when found with drug paraphernalia, and obvious signs of intoxication.

Adverse Psychological Effects

Cannabis produces effects on cognition, affect, and anxiety and can alter perceptions, leading to hallucinations or paranoia. Several neuropsychological changes and deficits have been identified with marijuana intoxication as well as long-term use; dose-dependent cognitive changes can persist up to 1 month after initiating abstinence (Bolla et al. 2002). Performance decrements in complex reaction time tasks, digit code memory tasks, fine motor function, time estimation, ability to track information over time, tactual form discrimination, and concept formation have been found. These impairments are proportional to use, last for some time beyond intoxication, and may be due to regional brain injury to the amygdala and hippocampus (Yücel et al. 2008). This translates into impairment in automobile driving, airplane flying, or any other complex motor skill. Impaired attention span, coordination, and depth perception have been found 10 hours or more after use. Undesirable physical effects include conjunctivitis, dry mouth, and light-headedness.

In terms of emotional responses, it is notable that anxiety, confusion, fear, and increased dependency can progress to panic or frank paranoid pathology. Marijuana also can exacerbate depression and has been found to increase the risk of developing depressive symptoms, even in prospective studies (Bovasso 2001). Epidemiological studies have demonstrated that cannabis dependence is associated with a heightened risk for suicidal ideation and suicide attempts (Lynskey et al. 2004). As described in Chapter 5 ("Definition, Presentation, and Diagnosis"), a syndrome of cannabis withdrawal has been established.

Psychosocial Function

Heavy users of cannabis have tended to report lower educational attainment and income, and differences have been shown to persist even after adjustment for many potentially confounding variables (Gruber et al. 2003). A behavioral profile associated with chronic cannabis use—amotivational syndrome—has been described (Grinspoon and Bakalar 2005). This concept characterizes people who become passive and decreasingly goal-directed and evidence declining drive, memory, and problem-solving ability with chronic marijuana use. Fatigue, apathy, and what has been described as a "fog" can last for several weeks after cessation of use. Amotivational syndrome has been controversial because of methodological problems in the research. It has been described most frequently in third-world countries, where environmental factors or preexisting personality factors may play a large role.

Relationship With Psychosis

Understanding of the relationship between psychosis and cannabis has been controversial for some time, although current understanding is that cannabis does not cause schizophrenia. On the other hand, persons with schizophrenia may be more likely to use cannabis, and the various psychic and neural stressors associated with cannabis may uncover an underlying psychotic process or vulnerability. The rates of psychiatric disorders of family members of persons both with cannabis-induced psychotic disorder and schizophrenia spectrum disorders were shown to be of the same magnitude (Arendt et al. 2008). Looking from a different perspective, patients with first-episode schizophrenia who use cannabis have been shown to have a more pronounced brain volume reduction than those not using, which is a stark effect of this substance (Rais et al. 2008).

Adverse Physical Effects

There is increasing evidence that marijuana abuse creates at least some long-term adverse physical effects. For example, several biochemical findings on physical effects have been reported. Marijuana has been studied in relationship to human male and female fertility, cell metabolism and protein synthesis, normal cell division, and spermatogenesis. Cannabis smoke contains carcinogens similar to tobacco smoke, and chronic marijuana abuse may predispose an individual to chronic obstructive lung disease and pulmonary neoplasm. Cannabis also increases heart rate and blood pressure, which may be crucial in patients with cardiovascular disease. Chronic marijuana abuse may lead to gynecomastia in males. The nonpsychological effects of cannabis, such as decreased fertility, increased lung problems (including cancer), and increased periodontal disease, might be helpful in motivating users to quit.

A final word about "medical" usage of marijuana: there are numerous conditions for which marijuana has been suggested as a therapeutic agent. An Institute of Medicine (1999) report recommends compassionate use of marijuana products for debilitating medical conditions such as HIV and cancer. Individuals with multiple sclerosis who smoke "street" cannabis tend to have more extensive cognitive abnormalities compared with those who do not (Ghaffar and Feinstein 2008). Further research is needed in this area.

Nicotine

Course

Like addiction with other substances of abuse, tobacco addiction frequently presents as a relapsing condition. Cigarette experimentation usually begins in the teenage years. Environmental influences are important; factors such as peer tobacco use (both in youth and in adults), parental tobacco use, and use of other substances contribute to initiation and maintenance of use. Various nonpharmacological aspects of smoking, such as social aspects, relief of boredom, and effect on self-image, may actively account for some of the reinforcing behavior in which dependent smokers engage.

Among those who attempt to quit, relapse may be evident during periods of high stress, anxiety or maladjustment, poor social support, or low self-confidence. There is a strong association between alcohol and smoking. Frequently, alcoholics are able to stop drinking but have great difficulty giving up smoking at the same time. Many alcohol treatment programs essentially ignore the tobacco addiction; however, tobacco is a major health risk in this population and should be addressed at some point in treatment.

Factors associated with poor long-term outcome consist of poor overall adjustment, inadequate social support, environmental stress, being around people who continue to smoke, being uninformed about the dangers of cigarette smoking, dual diagnosis, and having a high level of use or tolerance. Notwithstanding interest in genetic vulnerability to nicotine, other findings have demonstrated the association between certain adverse experiences in childhood and smoking during adolescence and adulthood. Early initiation, current smoking, and heavy smoking—all are associated with a history of emotional abuse, sexual abuse, physical abuse, and other adverse conditions (Anda et al. 1999).

Quit Attempts

Only 33% of "self-quitters" are abstinent after 2 days. Around 80% of current smokers report having tried to quit. Less than 5% succeed more than 12 months on any quit attempt, which is defined by research criteria as stopping for 1 day. But each smoker makes repeated quit attempts and, over time, more than one-half are able to stop, with an average of seven attempts. Through the latter half of the twentieth century, most who quit did so without assistance (Marlatt et al. 1988). To the extent that quit rates with nicotine replacement therapies, various medications, or other support are not absolute, there is a basis for the concept that smoking is more complicated than nicotine use alone would suggest. Around 75%–80% of quitters relapse within 1 month. It is a "lengthy, demanding, and often-frustrating undertaking" (U.S. Department of Health and Human Services 2000). Positive self-efficacy and motivation are important predictors of positive prognostic indicators. Patients are often successful at quitting once they contract a serious illness such as heart disease or cancer. Women are often motivated and successful at stopping smoking when pregnant and are eager to protect the fetus. Quitting at any point along the way helps reduce the harmful effects of smoking. Nicotine decreases the effectiveness of chemotherapeutic agents for lung cancer, and stopping smoking helps to prevent recurrence of cancer illness.

Adverse Medical Sequelae

Tobacco remains the leading preventable cause of death in the United States. There is growing evidence of its dose-dependent link to cataracts in men. Nicotine tends to increase liver drug metabolism and therefore may lower the levels of medications metabolized by the liver. Psychotropic medications, including antipsychotics and antidepressants, may have lower blood levels in smokers. Stopping smoking is strongly recommended during pregnancy because smoking is associated with low birth weight and increased toxicity to the fetus. Clinicians should also be aware of the possibility that smoking is a risk for dementia at older ages (Sabia et al. 2008).

Inhalants

Course

Inhalant users are predominantly socially and economically deprived young males, ages 13–15 years. American and Mexican Indians and teenagers in the Southwest have been found to have a high prevalence of inhalant use. Amyl nitrite was popular in the 1970s in the homosexual population and continues to be used. Nitrous oxide use may be prevalent among certain health personnel, especially dentists. Most users tend to cease the use after a relatively short period of time and may go on to abuse other psychoactive substances. There is a fairly strong association between aggressive, disruptive, and antisocial behavior and inhalant intoxication.

Adverse Medical Effects

Deaths due to inhalants have been reported and appear to result from central respiratory depression, cardiac arrhythmia, and accidents. Long-term damage to bone marrow, kidneys, liver, neuromuscular tissue, and brain has been reported.

Key Points

- Earlier use of a substance is associated with not only a more complicated and severe addiction but also with a greater likelihood of abuse of other substances and high-risk behaviors.
- Use of drugs or alcohol is associated with long-term cognitive, psychological, and medical problems, and can be damaging to a developing fetus.
- Early detection and treatment are essential to preventing and minimizing the long-term negative consequences of substance abuse.

References

American Academy of Pediatrics Committee on Drugs: Neonatal drug withdrawal. Pediatrics 101:1079–1088, 1998

Anda RF, Croft, JB, Felitti, VJ, et al: Adverse childhood experiences and smoking during adolescence and adulthood. JAMA 282:1652–1658, 1999

Arendt M, Mortensen PB, Rosenberg R, et al: Familial predisposition for psychiatric disorder: comparison of subjects treated for cannabis-induced psychosis and schizophrenia. Arch Gen Psychiatry 65:1269–1274, 2008

Armor DJ, Polish SM, Stambul HB: Alcoholics and Treatment. New York, Wiley, 1978

Bolla KI, Brown K, Eldreth D, et al: Dose-related neurocognitive effects of marijuana use. Neurology 59:1337–1343, 2002

Bovasso GB: Cannabis abuse as a risk factor for depressive symptoms. Am J Psychiatry 158:2033–2037, 2001

Caplan JP, Epstein LA, Quinn DK, et al: Neuropsychiatric effects of prescription drug abuse. Neuropsychol Rev 17:363–380, 2007

Cloninger CR, Sigvardsson S, Bohman M: Type I and type II alcoholism: an update. Alcohol Health and Research World 20:18–23, 1996

Crews FT, Buckley T, Dodd PR, et al: Alcoholic neurobiology: changes in dependence and recovery. Alcohol Clin Exp Res 29:1504–1513, 2005

Gallop RJ, Crits-Christoph P, Ten Have TR, et al: Differential transitions between cocaine use and abstinence for men and women. J Consult Clin Psychol 75:95–103, 2007

Ghaffar O, Feinstein A: Multiple sclerosis and cannabis: a cognitive and psychiatric study. Neurology 71:164–169, 2008

Grinspoon L, Bakalar JB: Marihuana, in Substance Abuse: Clinical Problems and Perspectives, 4th Edition. Edited by Lowinson JL, Ruiz P, Millman RB, et al. Baltimore, MD, Williams & Wilkins, 2005, pp 263–276

Gruber AJ, Pope HG, Hudson JI, et al: Attributes of long-term heavy cannabis users: a case-control study. Psychol Med 33:1415–1422, 2003

Henwood B, Padgett DK: Reevaluating the self-medication hypothesis among the dually diagnosed. Am J Addict 16:160–165, 2007

Hingson RW, Heeren T, Winter MR: Age at drinking onset and alcohol dependence: age at onset, duration, and severity. Arch Pediatr Adolesc Med 160:739–746, 2006

Institute of Medicine, Division of Neuroscience and Behavioral Health: Marijuana and Medicine: Assessing the Science Base. Edited by Joy JE, Watson SJ Jr, Benson JA Jr. Washington, DC, National Academy Press, 1999

Jellinek EM: The Disease Concept of Alcoholism. New Haven, CT, Hillhouse Press, 1960

Kandel D, Faust R: Sequence and stages in patterns of adolescent drug use. Arch Gen Psychiatry 32:923–932, 1975

Karch DL, Lubell KM, Friday J, et al: Surveillance for violent deaths—National Violent Death Reporting System, 16 states, 2005. MMWR Surveill Summ 57:1–45, 2008

Khantzian EJ: The self-medication hypothesis of substance use disorders: a reconsideration and recent applications. Harv Rev Psychiatry 4:231–244, 1997

Kranzler HR, Armeli S, Feinn R, et al: Targeted naltrexone treatment moderates the relations between mood and drinking behavior among problem drinkers. J Consult Clin Psychol 72:317–327, 2004

Lieber CS: Medical disorders of alcoholism. N Engl J Med 333:1058–1065, 1995

Lynskey MT, Heath AC, Bucholz KK, et al: Escalation of drug use in early-onset cannabis users vs. co-twin controls. JAMA 289:427–433, 2003

Lynskey MT, Glowinski AL, Todorov AA, et al: Major depressive disorder, suicidal ideation, and suicide attempt in twins discordant for cannabis dependence and early onset cannabis use. Arch Gen Psychiatry 61:1026–1032, 2004

Marlatt GA, Curry S, Gordon JR: A longitudinal analysis of unaided smoking cessation. Clin Cons Psychol 56:715–720, 1988

McCarty CA, Ebel BE, Garrison MM, et al: Continuity of binge and harmful drinking from late adolescence to early adulthood. Pediatrics 114:714–719, 2004

Nanda A, Vannemreddy P, Willis B, et al: Stroke in the young: relationship of active cocaine use with stroke mechanism and outcome. Acta Neurochir Suppl 96:91–96, 2006

Rais M, Cahn W, Van Haren N, et al: Excessive brain volume loss over time in cannabis-using first-episode schizophrenia patients. Am J Psychiatry 165:490–496, 2008

Sabia S, Marmot M, Dufouil C, et al: Smoking history and cognitive function in middle age from the Whitehall II study. Arch Intern Med 168:1165–1173, 2008

Schuckit MA, Smith TL, Danko GP, et al: Five-year clinical course associated with DSM-IV alcohol abuse or dependence in a large group of men and women. Am J Psychiatry 158:1084–1090, 2001

Sekine Y, Ouchi Y, Takei N, et al: Brain serotonin transporter density and aggression in abstinent methamphetamine users. Arch Gen Psychiatry 63:90–100, 2006

Spiehler VR, Reed D: Brain concentrations of cocaine and benzoylecgonine in fatal cases. J Forensic Sci 30:1003–1011, 1985

U.S. Department of Health and Human Services: Reducing Tobacco Use: A Report of the Surgeon General. Atlanta, GA, Centers for Disease Control and Prevention, National Center for Chronic Disease Prevention and Health Promotion, Office on Smoking and Health, 2000

Vaillant GE: A long-term follow-up of male alcohol abuse. Arch Gen Psychiatry 53:243–249, 1996

Volkow ND, Wang GJ, Fowler JS, et al: Stimulant-induced enhanced sexual desire as a potential contributing factor in HIV transmission. Am J Psychiatry 164:157–160 2007

Wang GJ, Volkow N, Chang L, et al: Partial recovery of brain metabolism in methamphetamine abusers after protracted abstinence. Am J Psychiatry161:242–248, 2004

Yücel M, Solowij N, Respondek C, et al: Regional brain abnormalities associated with long-term heavy cannabis use. Arch Gen Psychiatry 65:694–701, 2008

7

Violence and Suicide, Injury, Corrections, and Forensics

Injuries, violence, suicide, interpersonal conflicts, lawsuits, psychiatric commitment, or even crimes (and sentences) are often a part of the lives of those who misuse substances.

Violence and Crime

Violence

Substance use has been linked with both aggression and violence (including suicide) (Hoaken and Stewart 2003), independent of crime and incarceration. Earlier expression of conduct disorder portends a higher rate of substance use and vice versa, and individuals with antisocial personality disorder are 21 times as likely to develop alcohol abuse or dependence at some point in their lives (Moeller and Dougherty 2001). This relationship is not limited to alcohol; it is present in nicotine, cocaine, amphetamine, and cannabis use (Tardiff et al. 1994; Budney et al. 2004). Risk of violence among the severely mentally ill does not usually exceed that of the general population, except when there is co-occurring substance use (Swartz et al. 1998). The risk of perpetration of both intimate-partner violence and child maltreatment (Schuck and Widom 2003) increases with substances of abuse. Treatment is effective: risk of intimate-partner violence has been shown to be reduced following outpatient treatment of the male alcoholic partner (O'Farrell et al. 2003) or following structured behavioral couples therapy (O'Farrell et al. 2004).

Crime

The association between substance use and crime is also well established (Grann and Fazel 2004), and frequency of criminal behavior increases with the severity of substance use. Of people arrested for violent offenses, 70% test positive for substances (Sinha and Easton 1999). Cannabis use is associated with crimes involving weapons and crimes such as reckless endangerment and attempted homicide (Friedman et al. 2001). Among women, serious violent offending is correlated with misuse of alcohol, alcohol and cocaine together, or cannabis (J.A. Phillips et al. 2002).

Suicide

The use of substances is associated with suicide. In some cases, this association exists because of a confluence of depressed mood, substance use, and suicidal thoughts. But for alcohol, nicotine, and cocaine, there is a risk of suicide independent of any underlying or "co-occurring" non–substance induced psychiatric disorder (Harris and Barraclough 1997). According to a 2004 World Health Organization study, substance-use-related disorders are involved in 17% of completed suicides (Bertolote et al. 2004). A carefully performed data reanalysis indicated that the lifetime suicide risk for individuals with affective disorders, alcoholism, and schizophrenia was 6%, 7%, and 4%, respectively (Inskip et al. 1998). There are many psychological and pathophysiological pathways by which substance use might affect suicidality (Table 7–1). Data on the role of specific substances and other factors in suicide are described in the following subsections.

Table 7–1. Substance-induced contributors to suicidality

Short-term

Disinhibition (dose dependent)

Agitation

Psychosis (e.g., "bad trips")

Impulsivity

Irritability

Depression

Violence

Overdose

Physiological withdrawal

Hopelessness

Long-term

CNS injury (especially to frontal lobes)

Medical illness, injuries

Social stressors: illegal behaviors, gambling debts, fraud, legal, social, occupational, accidents, arrests

Poor/estranged social supports

Tendency for "thrill-seeking behavior"

Past exposure to traumatic or violent situations

Note. CNS = central nervous system.

Alcohol

Alcohol use has a central role in suicides. Different retrospective and prospective investigations have demonstrated an excess suicide risk among alcohol users compared with both the general and non-substance-using psychiatric populations. Recent alcohol use increases suicide risk dramatically in comparison with abstinent individuals (Kolves et al. 2006). Factors predictive of suicide completion in alcohol misuse are listed in Table 7–2.

Opioids

The pharmacology of opioids impacts their ability to engender distress and any resulting suicidality, but withdrawal from opioids can be extremely dis-

Table 7–2.   Factors predictive of suicide completion in alcohol misuse

Heavy drinking behavior in days and months prior to suicide

Poor social support

Living alone

Talking to others about suicide

Serious medical consequences of alcohol

Being unemployed

Prior suicide attempts

Earlier onset of addiction

More severe dependence

Other substance dependence

Being separated or divorced

More likely to have had treatment

More panic symptoms, and more likely to have been diagnosed with a substance-induced psychiatric disorder

Source.   Adapted from Murphy et al. 1992; Preuss et al. 2003.

tressing. As noted later in this chapter (see "Sedatives/Hypnotics" subsection), misuse of prescription medications carries a great risk for suicide (Harris and Barraclough 1997). Among recovering opioid users being maintained on methadone, risk of suicide attempts was correlated with female gender, violent behavior in the past 30 days and over the lifetime, and less education, whereas current suicidal ideation was correlated with current family conflict and depression severity (J. Phillips et al. 2004). Relapse to opioid use poses the additional hazard of the lethality of overdose in those who are feeling suicidal.

Cocaine

The role of cocaine use in suicide should not be underestimated. Marzuk et al. (1992) found that 29% of suicide victims in New York ages 21–30 years tested positive for cocaine, and data from 13,673 participants in the Epidemiologic Catchment Area survey in the United States showed that cocaine abusers had a significantly greater risk of attempting suicide (Petronis et al. 1990). Characteristics of cocaine-dependent patients who attempted suicide are listed in Table 7–3 (Roy 2001).

Table 7–3. Factors associated with suicide attempts among cocaine users

Female gender
Family history of suicidal behavior
Reported childhood trauma
Introversion
Neuroticism
Hostility
Co-occurring alcohol dependence
Co-occurring opiate dependence
Co-occurring major depression
Co-occurring medical disorders

Source. Adapted from Roy 2001.

Inhalants

Suicide risk among those who use inhalants has been documented. Adolescents who have used inhalants (a group likely to be using other substances as well) tend to have had a significantly greater number of past suicide attempts than adolescents not using inhalants (Sakai et al. 2004).

Stimulants/Amphetamines, Hallucinogens, Ketamine/ Phencyclidine, and Gamma-Hydroxybutyrate

There is little literature on the convergence of use of stimulants/amphetamines, hallucinogens, ketamine/phencyclidine, and gamma-hydroxybutyrate substances with suicidality. But each may produce physiological disturbances that can be fatal, or they can produce either psychotic symptomatology or other states (see Table 7–1) that may lead to suicidal behavior.

Cannabis

There is increasing evidence that cannabis use is associated with antisocial behavior and violence (Brook et al. 2003). In the study by Harris and Barraclough (1997), cannabis users had a suicide risk 4 times that of nonusers.

Nicotine

There is an "unmistakable" dose-dependent association between nicotine use and suicide, which persists even after controlling for income, age, race, prior myocardial infarction, diabetes, alcohol use (Malone et al. 2003), and prior depression (Breslau et al. 2005; Wu et al. 2004). Nicotine withdrawal can be agitating.

Sedatives/Hypnotics

The risk of suicide among those misusing sedatives or hypnotics is significant. One study showed that the risks of suicide among those misusing prescribed medications included a relative risk of 20 with solely the misused medication, 16 with the medication and alcohol, and 114 with the medication and any illicit drug (Harris and Barraclough 1997)! The abuse of prescription medications in combination with alcohol or with illicit drugs carries with it an additive risk for accidental overdose.

Assessment and treatment of this group of patients should typically follow general guidelines for the management of suicidal or parasuicidal patients (American Academy of Child and Adolescent Psychiatry 2001; American Psychiatric Association 2003), but additional points should be emphasized. At the least, there are five essential components of the management of the substance-using individual with suicidality: 1) safety, 2) protection from significant withdrawal syndrome, 3) abstinence, 4) treatment of comorbid conditions, and 5) relapse prevention.

Unintentional Injury

In each U.S. age group from 1 through 44 years, deaths resulting from unintentional injuries exceed all other causes, including suicide (Centers for Disease Control and Prevention 2005), and, for many cases, this is associated with use of substances. Deaths may result from use of substances or from other activities while intoxicated; falls, traffic accidents, violence, and short- and long-term medical consequences are dangers associated with substances generally. The potential for accidental death by overdose varies by substance: high for opioids and barbiturates, lower for alcohol and benzodiazepines.

Even small amounts of alcohol (lower than the legal limit) can reduce perception of crash risk in partially sleep-deprived individuals. Such risks apply to use of any machinery, even bicycles. Cannabis is often implicated as well—one study demonstrated that among those causing auto crashes, 50%–80% of those who tested positive for cannabis also tested positive for alcohol (Ramaekers et al. 2004).

Correctional Settings

Correctional settings provide a platform for treatment that differs from the typical clinical situation. Both the American Psychiatric Association (2000) and the National Commission on Correctional Health Care (2003) have developed guidelines for correctional facilities, and the Office of Juvenile Justice and Delinquency Prevention (2004) has created guidelines for clinicians who come into contact with incarcerated youth.

There are three very different incarceration ecologies in which the individual exists: the lockup (upon arrest), jail (following arraignment, during trial, prior to sentencing, or in sentences of up to 1 year), and prison (post-sentencing, more than 1 year). Substance-related disorders may appear at any point in the correctional process.

Entry/Screening

Any drug of abuse may be present in the body of an individual when he or she enters custody directly from the outside world; many arrestees have been using just prior to arrest. This "intake" is a critical moment when the staff must look carefully for intoxication, overdose, medical complications, or active withdrawal from any substance—especially alcohol, benzodiazepines, or other sedatives.

Treatment and Rehabilitation

Substance use disorders (SUDs) in this population are often accompanied by a variety of other concerns, such as mental health issues, unemployment, and lack of education, which make successful treatment and recovery more difficult (Belenko and Peugh 2005).

Disposition After Discharge

On discharge, both those with SUDs and those with SUDs comorbid with psychiatric conditions are at high risk of relapse, which may affect criminality as well. Data suggest that psychosocial aspects of reentry are the most important in reducing relapse and recidivism (Rounds-Bryant et al. 2004). A National Institute on Drug Abuse (2006) guide is helpful for professionals working in these settings.

Mandated Treatment

Various jurisdictions—but not all—have developed systems for court authority to encourage, or to force, individuals into psychiatric or substance use care. The cascade of names and laws for these systems may be confusing. These provisions may overlap in some jurisdictions; they may have different names despite similar procedures and goals.

Criminal Diversion

"Diversion" refers to institutions, practices, and laws that divert criminal offenders who have a mental disorder or an SUD out of the standard criminal justice system and into alternatives. This may be done at many different points in the criminal process including pre-arrest, pre-arraignment, pretrial, in lieu of punishment, or after some punishment. The core feature of diversion is that an authority releases the offender from further blame or from punishment in return for engaging in treatment. Typically, the offender must demonstrate to the authority (police, prosecutor, or judge) a voluntary willingness to engage in treatment. Drug courts are one type of diversion that have led to low criminal recidivism rates and lead to education, cost savings, and babies being born drug-free.

Mandated Treatment/Commitment

Mandated treatment exists in some jurisdictions for those with serious and pervasive SUDs who have been or will likely become dangerous to themselves or others. Various states, counties, and the federal government have been developing ways in which to intervene (Gerbasi et al. 2000).

Forensic Practice

In any situation in which a clinician has been asked to respond specifically to the question(s) of an authority, the process by which that answer is created is as important as the content of the answer itself. The pieces of the process that are most important include those that ensure that the communication is consistent with the ideals of the American Academy of Psychiatry and the Law: 1) honesty and 2) striving for objectivity (American Academy of Psychiatry and the Law 2005). Although both clinical psychiatry and forensic psychiatry are based on solid knowledge of current medical knowledge and, when appropriate, careful assessment of the individual and his or her mental state, they differ in their goals. Forensic psychiatry is the provision of objective statements regarding psychiatric conditions for certain audiences that seek responses to specific questions. The forensic psychiatrist's need to eschew bias and "strive for objectivity" is disparate from the clinician's interest in altruistic clinical intervention and the clinician's method of communication with other clinicians.

Areas of Expertise in Forensic Addiction Practice

The opinion of the addiction expert may be desired by various parties in different forms of formal dispute resolution—this extends beyond criminal law to civil law, administrative proceedings, and diversion programs. In each state, laws define specific criteria that must be met as a part of an expert's opinion, and the expert must have a grasp of that legal language before engaging in any consultation.

Criminal Defense

Over time, case law and statutes have almost completely eliminated voluntary intoxication as a defense against responsibility. On the other hand, *involuntary* intoxication may be exculpatory. Also possibly exculpatory is "settled insanity," a situation in which long-term use has led to a chronic injury that is different from an acute intoxication or toxic psychosis. When "specific intent" is required for a person to be convicted of a particular charge, voluntary intoxication has been successfully used as a defense. In some states, the forensic psychiatrist may be asked to investigate the presence or absence of *mens rea* ("evil intent," a condition of the individual that must be proven in every criminal prosecution) when the substance was first ingested. In some situations, intoxication may directly implicate a defendant as guilty. Crimes such as driving while intoxicated (DWI) or driving under the influence (DUI) are called "strict liability crimes." For such charges, *mens rea* is not required for a conviction.

In some cases in which criminal or civil offenses have been alleged, the defendant who is an abuser of drugs or alcohol may state that he or she is not able to comment upon the act because he or she was in a state of "blackout." Forensic psychiatrists, especially those without much experience in addiction psychiatry, may misuse, inappropriately downplay, or otherwise misapply blackouts. Concerns about malingering have fed this doubt. However, addiction psychiatrists are familiar with blackouts as a clinical phenomenon, and their input to the court may be very helpful in related cases. It is important to distinguish this effect of intoxication from amnesia. Intoxication or other states secondary to substances may be invoked as the basis for being incapacitated at the time of *Miranda* warnings or during interrogation.

Criminal Sentencing Recommendations

In various jurisdictions, psychiatric opinions may be sought in the sentencing phase. The psychiatrist can wield great influence in identifying SUDs and making clear recommendations for treatment, both during a sentence and after the sentence would be completed. A case in the federal system, *United States v. Booker* (2005), provides leeway to U.S. District Court judges to diverge from sentencing guidelines if the presence of psychiatric (including substance use) disorders substantially affected some part of the criminal behavior.

Family and Matrimonial Law

In disputes over divorce, custody, guardianship, adoption, or child safety, the substance use of any involved party is commonly at issue. The fiercely adversarial nature of these proceedings often impedes the formation of a valid picture. Collateral sources of information may be helpful in clarifying central issues, such as what may be in the best interests of the child or children.

Personal Injury

Substance abuse issues often arise when an individual who is injured sues another party for damages. Either side may allege that the other was intoxicated at the time of the injury, and may seek the help of a psychiatrist to establish or to negate such claims. The impact of long-term addiction may also be raised. Injured parties may also blame the party that provides the substance of abuse. Sexual harassment cases may be brought in either criminal or civil settings, and addictions may be raised as an issue in such cases as well.

Disability

Claims of disability based on addictions may be made to private insurance companies or to the federal government. Addiction psychiatrists are naturally the experts of choice for such cases. They may be retained by the individual claiming disability or by the insurance company for an "independent medical exam." If the case goes to court, expert testimony will be included. Any physician who completes "paperwork" certifying disability should consider the possibility that he or she may be called to testify about his or her findings in court. Management of addictions in patients with chronic pain complaints is clinically complex; this complexity translates in the question to the expert of whether or not return to work is possible or what is the level of disability. It is often appropriate for the treating psychiatrist to refer a patient for consultation with an addiction psychiatrist or pain expert when faced with such a question. A new guideline from the American Academy of Psychiatry and the Law (2005) may be helpful.

Malpractice

A patient may allege that a physician caused him to become addicted to substances or that his physician was impaired by substances.

Testamentary Capacity

The presence of substance use is frequently a part of retrospective challenges to testamentary capacity (Shulman et al. 2005)

Administrative Law

There are cases in which military or other administrative law proceedings require psychiatric input about addiction. These include noncivil and noncriminal institutions such as athletic, security, licensing, or ethics bodies. Administrative bodies may seek evidence about a person's degree of substance use and its effect on his or her ability to perform their obligations.

Key Points

- Exposure to substances increases risk of violence, suicide, and injury independently of psychiatric condition.
- Substance use may contribute to different facets of suicidal behavior.
- Specific substance-using populations may be at higher risk of suicide than others, especially users of nicotine and alcohol.
- The first three considerations in care of a substance-using suicidal individual are safety, protection from significant withdrawal syndromes, and abstinence.
- Clinicians should be vigilant about unwanted efforts to misuse them as legal experts.

References

American Academy of Child and Adolescent Psychiatry: Practice parameter for the assessment and treatment of children and adolescents with suicidal behavior. J Am Acad Child Adolesc Psychiatry 40 (suppl 7):24S–51S, 2001

American Academy of Psychiatry and the Law. Ethics guidelines for the practice of forensic psychiatry. Adopted May 2005. Available at: http://www.aapl.org/pdf/ETHICSGDLNS.pdf. Accessed June 13, 2009.

American Psychiatric Association: Psychiatric Services in Jails and Prisons: A Task Force Report of the American Psychiatric Association, 2nd Edition. Washington DC, American Psychiatric Association, 2000

American Psychiatric Association: Practice guideline for the assessment and treatment of patients with suicidal behaviors. Am J Psychiatry 160 (suppl 11):1–60, 2003

Belenko S, Peugh J: Estimating drug treatment needs among state prison inmates. Drug Alcohol Depend 77:269–281, 2005

Bertolote JM, Fleischmann A, De Leo D, et al: Psychiatric diagnoses and suicide: revisiting the evidence. Crisis 25:147–155, 2004

Breslau N, Schultz LR, Johnson EO, et al: Smoking and the risk of suicidal behavior: a prospective study of a community sample. Arch Gen Psychiatry 62:328–334, 2005

Brook JS, Brook DW, Rosen Z, et al: Earlier marijuana use and later problem behavior in Colombian youths. J Am Acad Child Adolesc Psychiatry 42:485–492, 2003

Budney AJ, Hughes JR, Moore BA, et al: Review of the validity and significance of cannabis withdrawal syndrome. Am J Psychiatry 161:1967–1977, 2004

Centers for Disease Control and Prevention: LCWK2: deaths, percentage of total deaths, and death rates for the 15 leading causes of death in 10-year age groups, by race and sex: United States, 2002. Hyattsville, MD, National Center for Health Statistics, July 2005. Available at: http://www.cdc.gov/nchs/data/dvs/LCWK2_2002.pdf. Accessed June 13, 2009.

Friedman AS, Glassman K, Terras BA, et al: Violent behavior as related to use of marijuana and other drugs. J Addict Dis 20:49–72, 2001

Gerbasi J, Bonnie R, Binder R: Resource document on mandatory outpatient treatment. J Am Acad Psychiatry Law 28:127–144, 2000

Grann M, Fazel S: Substance misuse and violent crime: Swedish population study. BMJ 328:1233–1234, 2004

Harris EC, Barraclough B: Suicide as an outcome for mental disorders. Br J Psychiatry 170:205–228, 1997

Hoaken PNS, Stewart SH: Drugs of abuse and the elicitation of human aggressive behavior. Addict Behav 28:1533–1554, 2003

Inskip HM, Harris EC, Barraclough B: Lifetime risk of suicide for affective disorder, alcoholism and schizophrenia. Br J Psychiatry 172:35–37, 1998

Kolves K, Varnik A, Tooding LM, et al: The role of alcohol in suicide: a case-control psychological autopsy study. Psychol Med 36:923–930, 2006

Malone KM, Waternaux C, Haas GL, et al: Cigarette smoking, suicidal behavior, and serotonin function in major psychiatric disorders. Am J Psychiatry 160:773–779, 2003

Marzuk PM, Tardiff K, Leon AC, et al: Prevalence of cocaine use among residents of New York City who committed suicide during a one-year period. Am J Psychiatry 149:371–375, 1992

Moeller FG, Dougherty DM: Antisocial personality disorder, alcohol, and aggression. Alcohol Res Health 25:5–11, 2001

Murphy GE, Wetzel RD, Robins E, et al: Multiple risk factors predict suicide in alcoholism. Arch Gen Psychiatry 49:439–443, 1992

National Commission on Correctional Health Care: Standards for Health Services in Prisons. Chicago, IL, National Commission on Correctional Health Care, 2003

National Institute on Drug Abuse: Principles of Drug Abuse Treatment for Criminal Justice Populations: A Research-Based Guide (NIH Publ No 06-5316). 2006. Available at: http://www.nida.nih.gov/PDF/PODAT_CJ/PODAT_CJ.pdf. Accessed June 13, 2009.

O'Farrell TJ, Fals-Stewart W, Murphy M, et al: Partner violence before and after individually based alcoholic patients. J Consult Clin Psychol 71:92–102, 2003

O'Farrell TJ, Murphy CM, Stephan SH, et al: Partner violence before and after couples-based alcoholism treatment for male alcoholic patients. J Consult Clin Psychol 72:202–217, 2004

Office of Juvenile Justice and Delinquency Prevention: Screening and Assessing Mental Health and Substance Use Disorders Among Youth in the Juvenile Justice System: A Resource Guide for Practitioners (NCJ 204956). Washington, DC, National Center for Mental Health and Juvenile Justice, December 2004. Available at: http://www.ncjrs.org/pdffiles1/ojjdp/204956.pdf. Accessed June 13, 2009.

Petronis K, Samuels J, Moscicki E, et al: An epidemiologic investigation of potential risk factors for suicide attempts. Soc Psychiatry Psychiatr Epidemiol 25:193–199, 1990

Phillips J, Carpenter KM, Nunes EV: Suicide risk in depressed methadone-maintained patients: associations with clinical and demographic characteristics. Am J Addict 13:327–332, 2004

Phillips JA, Nixon SJ, Pfefferbaum B: A comparison of substance abuse among female offender subtypes. J Am Acad Psychiatry Law 30:513–519, 2002

Preuss UW, Schuckit MA, Smith TL, et al: Predictors and correlates of suicide attempts over 5 years in 1,237 alcohol-dependent men and women. Am J Psychiatry 160:56–63, 2003

Ramaekers JG, Berghaus G, van Laar M, et al: Dose related risk of motor vehicle crashes after cannabis use. Drug Alcohol Depend 73:109–119, 2004

Rounds-Bryant JL, Motivans MA, Pelissier BM: Correlates of drug treatment outcomes for African American and white male federal prisoners: results from the TRIAD study. Am J Drug Alcohol Abuse 30:495–514, 2004

Roy A: Characteristics of cocaine-dependent patients who attempt suicide. Am J Psychiatry 158:1215–1219, 2001

Sakai JT, Hall SK, Mikulich-Gilbertson SK, et al: Inhalant use, abuse, and dependence among adolescent patients: commonly comorbid problems. J Am Acad Child Adolesc Psychiatry 43:1080–1088, 2004

Schuck AM, Widom CS: Childhood victimization and alcohol symptoms in women: an examination of protective factors. J Stud Alcohol 64:247–256, 2003

Shulman KI, Cohen CA, Hull I: Psychiatric issues in retrospective challenges of testamentary capacity. Int J Geriatr Psychiatry 20:63–69, 2005

Sinha R, Easton C: Substance abuse and criminality. J Am Acad Psychiatry Law 27:513–526, 1999

Swartz MS, Swanson JW, Hiday VA, et al: Violence and severe mental illness: the effects of substance abuse and nonadherence to medication. Am J Psychiatry 155:226–231, 1998

Tardiff K, Marzuk PM, Leon AC, et al: Homicide in New York City. Cocaine use and firearms. JAMA 272:43–46, 1994

United States v Booker, 543 U.S. 220 (2005)

Wu P, Hoven CW, Liu X, et al; Substance use, suicidal ideation and attempts in children and adolescents. Suicide Life Threat Behav 34:408–420, 2004

8

Behavioral Addictions

Among the disorders in DSM-IV-TR (American Psychiatric Association 2000), some have been described as "behavioral addictions," and the literature supports that they are addictions similar to those for physical substances. Specific disorders such as pathological gambling and kleptomania are included in DSM-IV-TR and have specific criteria sets. However, they are not included in DSM-IV-TR as addictive disorders, and the generic DSM-IV-TR criteria for the various substance use disorders (SUDs) do not apply to these behavioral conditions. Some have theorized that these conditions represent disorders of compulsion (such as obsessive-compulsive disorder), but at this point there is greater weight in viewing them from the standpoint of addictions. Criteria have been proposed for other uncontrolled behaviors, including compulsive computer use, compulsive sexual behavior, and compulsive buying (American Psychiatric Association 2000), but the literature is sparse with regard to those conditions. Notwithstanding their status in the diagnostic manual, when they do present to clinicians, patients with these conditions often seek addiction specialists. The frequent comorbidity of these conditions with other SUDs heightens the need for awareness of their impact and the necessity of treatment for them.

Basis of Overlap Among Addictions

The overlap among these conditions mostly lies in similar phenomenology. The literature recognizes that behavioral addictions and substance addictions share certain features:

- Repetitive or compulsive engagement in a behavior (e.g., gambling or exposing one's body to a substance) despite adverse consequences
- Impairment in major areas of life functioning (Blanco et al. 2002)
- Diminished control over the problematic behavior
- An urge or craving state prior to the problematic behavior
- A euphoric (or, at the least, euthymic) sensation during the performance of the problematic behavior or intoxication with the substance

Comorbidity between pathological gambling and SUDs and among the SUDS is another contributor to the overlap: epidemiological data indicate high rates of co-occurrence in each direction (Potenza et al. 2002), and high rates of both pathological gambling and SUDs have been reported during adolescence and young adulthood (Barnes et al. 2009). Finally, the behavioral addictions often respond to clinical interventions, including medications, as a means to curtail or eradicate the problem.

Epidemiology

The literature on the epidemiology of pathological gambling is large and perhaps as good as that of any of the other impulse-control disorders (Potenza et al. 2001; Kessler et al. 2008). It is estimated that the lifetime prevalence of pathological gambling among adults ranges from 0.9% to 1.6% and that past-year rates range from 0.6% to 1.1% (Grant and Potenza 2008). Like the SUDs, high levels of gambling and pathological gambling occur in males, especially in adolescence and young adulthood. Although the prevalence of kleptomania remains unknown, an estimate of 0.6% has been reported (Grant and Kim 2002). Estimates of the lifetime prevalence of compulsive buying have ranged from 1.8% to 6.0% (Koran et al. 2006).

Etiology and Neurobiology

In addition to genetic and familial factors, the current approach to the biological etiology of the behavioral addictions includes the understanding of the impulse-control disorders, in which multiple neurotransmitter systems (e.g., serotonergic, dopaminergic, noradrenergic, opioidergic) contribute. The serotonin system is thought to underlie impulse control. Imaging studies have also demonstrated findings during "withdrawal" from the various problem behaviors (Potenza 2008).

Pathological Gambling

Clinical Characteristics and Natural History

It is significant that, like SUDs, pathological gambling is defined as "chronic and persisting" (Slutske 2006) (see Table 8–1 for DSM-IV-TR diagnostic criteria). As a behavior, gambling usually begins during youth and at an earlier age for males than for females (Barnes et al. 2009). Higher rates of pathological gambling are observed in men, with shortening ("telescoping") of the progression to addiction observed in females (Dannon et al. 2006); and there are increased rates of pathological gambling in adolescents and young adults. In addition, individuals with pathological gambling tend to display some cognitive deficits, particularly in the temporal discounting of rewards and in the poor performance on decision-making tasks, which may be related to the behavior of gambling itself (Grant and Kim 2001). Large epidemiological surveys have found that "natural" recovery occurs in roughly one-third of all affected individuals (Kessler et al. 2008).

Co-Occurring Disorders

It is essential to be aware of the other psychiatric disorders with which the behavioral addictions are frequently comorbid, including mood, anxiety, and personality disorders. Indeed, in terms of lifetime prevalence, individuals presenting with pathological gambling often have disorders of mood (60%–76%), anxiety (16%–40%), or personality (87%), especially antisocial personality disorder. Furthermore, there often exist additional impulse-control disorders such as "compulsive" sexual behavior and intermittent explosive dis-

Table 8–1.   DSM-IV-TR diagnostic criteria for pathological gambling

A.   Persistent and recurrent maladaptive gambling behavior as indicated by five (or more) of the following:

   (1)   is preoccupied with gambling (e.g., preoccupied with reliving past gambling experiences, handicapping or planning the next venture, or thinking of ways to get money with which to gamble)

   (2)   needs to gamble with increasing amounts of money in order to achieve the desired excitement

   (3)   has repeated unsuccessful efforts to control, cut back, or stop gambling

   (4)   is restless or irritable when attempting to cut down or stop gambling

   (5)   gambles as a way of escaping from problems or of relieving a dysphoric mood (e.g., feelings of helplessness, guilt, anxiety, depression)

   (6)   after losing money gambling, often returns another day to get even ("chasing" one's losses)

   (7)   lies to family members, therapist, or others to conceal the extent of involvement with gambling

   (8)   has committed illegal acts such as forgery, fraud, theft, or embezzlement to finance gambling

   (9)   has jeopardized or lost a significant relationship, job, or educational or career opportunity because of gambling

   (10)   relies on others to provide money to relieve a desperate financial situation caused by gambling

B.   The gambling behavior is not better accounted for by a manic episode.

order (Bechara 2003). In terms of SUDs, alcohol use disorders are the disorders most often comorbid with pathological gambling (Liu et al. 2009). Moreover, the frequent co-occurrence of pathological gambling and nicotine use is often overlooked. Any comorbid use of substances that affect judgment can impair the individual's successful navigation away from gambling. By definition, mania or bipolar disorder is mutually exclusive with pathological gambling and would take diagnostic precedence over pathological gambling if they appeared to be comorbid.

Treatment

Both medications and psychosocial therapies are used for pathological gambling. Helpful medications include the antidepressants—particularly the serotonin reuptake inhibitors (especially fluvoxamine) and the tricyclic antidepressant clomipramine—and the opioid antagonists naltrexone (which is frequently employed in impulse-control disorders; el-Guebaly et al. 2006) and nalmefene (Leung and Cottler 2009). In terms of psychosocial therapies, most have some cognitive or behavioral basis. Cognitive-behavioral therapy has also been used to prevent (Doiron and Nicki 2007) and treat pathological gambling (Grant et al. 2006). Many gamblers benefit from Gamblers Anonymous and other 12-Step approaches, especially when comorbidity is present. Brief interventions also have been studied (Petry et al. 2008). Aversion therapy has shown positive outcomes in studies.

Kleptomania

Clinical Characteristics and Natural History

Although it had been a part of the lexicon for some time, kleptomania was not included in DSM until the publication of DSM-III (American Psychiatric Association 1980). Kleptomania's features include the recurrent (not sporadic) failure to resist the impulse to steal objects that are not needed for personal use or for their monetary value, an increasing sense of tension immediately before committing the theft, and the experience of pleasure, gratification, or release at the time of committing the theft. The stealing is not performed out of anger, vengeance, or due to psychosis, and it is not better accounted for by mania, antisocial personality disorder, or conduct disorder (American Psychiatric Association 2000). These criteria were crafted to ensure that the caseness did not include all robbers/shoplifters/burglars, but rather a specified group. One can see it includes similarities to compulsions generally. Like pathological gambling, kleptomania usually first appears during late adolescence or early adulthood. The course is generally chronic, with waxing and waning of activity. In terms of distribution by sex, there is a 2:1 ratio of women to men (Grant and Potenza 2008). Most individuals with kleptomania try to stop but tend not to be successful.

Co-Occurring Disorders and Family History

Concurrent diagnosis of other psychiatric disorders is high among persons with kleptomania, including the following diagnoses:

- Nonbipolar affective disorders: 59% (Grant and Kim 2002) to 100% (McElroy et al. 1991)
- Bipolar disorder: 9% (Grant and Kim 2002) to 60% (McElroy et al. 1991)
- Anxiety disorders: 60%–80% (McElroy et al. 1991)
- Impulse-control disorders: 20%–46% (Grant 2003)
- SUDs: 23%–50% (Grant and Kim 2002)
- Eating disorders: 60% (McElroy et al. 1991)

Furthermore, there is a higher-than-normal degree of family Axis I psychopathology among individuals with kleptomania (Grant 2003), particularly in terms of mood disorders (20%–35%) and SUDs (15%–20%) (McElroy et al. 1991).

Treatment

Effecting intervention for kleptomania requires ongoing attention, but there is little information to guide specific treatment. Medications that have been found effective include fluoxetine, nortriptyline, trazodone, clonazepam, valproate, lithium, fluvoxamine, paroxetine, and topiramate (Grant et al. 2009). The opioid antagonist naltrexone (dosages of 50–150 mg/day) has been shown in various studies to effect a significant decline in the intensity of urges to steal, thoughts of stealing, and stealing behavior (Grant et al. 2009). Although many psychotherapies have been applied to the treatment of kleptomania, the literature lacks controlled trials. Types of psychotherapy described in case reports as demonstrating success include psychoanalytic, insight-oriented, and behavioral (McElroy et al. 1991).

Compulsive Buying

Compulsive buying is not included in DSM-IV-TR. The proposed criteria (McElroy et al. 1994) include the following features:

- A maladaptive preoccupation with or engagement in buying (evidenced by frequent preoccupation with or irresistible impulses to buy; or frequent buying of items that are not needed or not affordable; or shopping for longer periods of time than intended).
- The preoccupations or the buying lead to significant distress or impairment.
- The buying does not occur exclusively during hypomanic or manic episodes.

As with other impulse-control disorders, compulsive buying first develops in late adolescence or early adulthood (Koran et al. 2006). Women more often present with compulsive buying, with some evidence pointing to a percentage exceeding 80% in clinical settings (Koran et al. 2006).

Key Points

- Many behavioral addictions, such as pathological gambling, kleptomania, and compulsive buying, have clinical characteristics that are similar to those of SUDs.
- The behavioral addictions are associated with significant impairment and distress.
- Individuals presenting with a behavioral addiction should be thoroughly assessed for comorbid substance use conditions and other Axis I psychiatric disorders.
- Both pharmacological and behavioral treatments are currently used for process addictions.

References

American Psychiatric Association: Diagnostic and Statistical Manual of Mental Disorders, 3rd Edition. Washington, DC, American Psychiatric Association, 1980

American Psychiatric Association: Diagnostic and Statistical Manual of Mental Disorders, 4th Edition, Text Revision. Washington, DC, American Psychiatric Association, 2000

Barnes GM, Welte JW, Hoffman JH, et al: Gambling, alcohol, and other substance use among youth in the United States. J Stud Alcohol Drugs 70:134–142, 2009

Bechara A: Risky business: emotion, decision-making, and addiction. J Gambl Stud 19:23–51, 2003

Blanco C, Petkova E, Ibanez A, et al: A pilot placebo-controlled study of fluvoxamine for pathological gambling. Ann Clin Psychiatry 14:9–15, 2002

Dannon PN, Lowengrub K, Shalgi B, et al: Dual psychiatric diagnosis and substance abuse in pathological gamblers: a preliminary gender comparison study. J Addict Dis 25:49–54, 2006

Doiron JP, Nicki RM: Prevention of pathological gambling: a randomized controlled trial. Cogn Behav Ther 36:74–84, 2007

el-Guebaly N, Patten SB, Currie S, et al: Epidemiological associations between gambling behavior, substance use and mood and anxiety disorders. J Gambl Stud 22:275–287, 2006

Grant JE: Family history and psychiatric comorbidity in persons with kleptomania. Compr Psychiatry 44:437–441, 2003

Grant JE, Kim SW: Demographic and clinical features of 131 adult pathological gamblers. J Clin Psychiatry 62:957–962, 2001

Grant JE, Kim SW: Clinical characteristics and associated psychopathology of 22 patients with kleptomania. Compr Psychiatry 43:378–384, 2002

Grant JE, Potenza MN: Gender-related differences in individuals seeking treatment for kleptomania. CNS Spectr 13:235–245, 2008

Grant JE, Potenza MN, Hollander E, et al: Multicenter investigation of the opioid antagonist nalmefene in the treatment of pathological gambling. Am J Psychiatry 163:303–312, 2006

Grant JE, Kim SW, Odlaug BL: A double-blind, placebo-controlled study of the opiate antagonist, naltrexone, in the treatment of kleptomania. Biol Psychiatry 65:600–606, 2009

Kessler RC, Hwang I, LaBrie R, et al: DSM-IV pathological gambling in the National Comorbidity Survey Replication. Psychol Med 38:1351–1360, 2008

Koran LM, Faber RJ, Aboujaoude E, et al: Estimated prevalence of compulsive buying behavior in the United States. Am J Psychiatry 163:1806–1812, 2006

Leung KS, Cottler LB: Treatment of pathological gambling. Curr Opin Psychiatry 22:69–74, 2009

Liu T, Maciejewski PK, Potenza MN: The relationship between recreational gambling and substance abuse/dependence: data from a nationally representative sample. Drug Alcohol Depend 100:164–168, 2009

McElroy SL, Pope HG, Hudson JI, et al: Kleptomania: a report of 20 cases. Am J Psychiatry 148:652–657, 1991

McElroy SL, Keck PE, Pope HG, et al: Compulsive buying: a report of 20 cases. J Clin Psychiatry 55:242–248, 1994

Petry NM, Weinstock J, Ledgerwood DM: A randomized trial of brief interventions for problem and pathological gamblers. J Consult Clin Psychol 76:318–328, 2008

Potenza MN: The neurobiology of pathological gambling and drug addiction: an overview and new findings. Philos Trans R Soc Lond B Biol Sci 363:3181–3189, 2008

Potenza MN, Kosten TR, Rounsaville BJ: Pathological gambling. JAMA 286:141–144, 2001

Potenza MN, Fiellin DA, Heninger GA, et al: Gambling: an addictive behavior with health and primary care implications. J Gen Intern Med 17:721–732, 2002

Slutske WS: Natural recovery and treatment-seeking in pathological gambling: results of two U.S. national surveys. Am J Psychiatry 163:297–302, 2006

9

Children and Adolescents

The use, abuse, prevention, and treatment of substance use disorders (SUDs) in children and adolescents are of grave concern, not least because their prevalence is rising, the age of first use is falling, and the morbidity and mortality associated with SUDs in youth are increasing. Substance abuse can interfere with natural growth and normal interaction and development, including relationships with peers, performance in school, attitudes toward law and authority, and acute and chronic organic effects. The question of when use becomes abuse and dependency in adolescents is controversial. There is a continuum between hazardous, harmful use and abuse. It is more difficult to diagnose dependence in adolescents because of the reduced likelihood of signs and symptoms of withdrawal that frequently occur later in addiction. Adolescents are less likely to report withdrawal symptoms, have shorter periods of addiction, and may recover more rapidly from withdrawal symptoms. Early identification of patterns of drug use that interfere with relationships, school performance, and ability to provide good self-care, in addition to physiological symptoms of tolerance and withdrawal, are important. There are specific practice parameters for the treatment of SUDs in children and adolescents (American Academy of Child and Adolescent Psychiatry 1997).

145

Extent of the Problem

As described in Chapter 2 ("Magnitude of the Problem"), substance use among children and adolescents remains a significant problem. Results of the Monitoring the Future study for 2008 showed that overall illicit drug use by teens was generally declining except for cannabis use, which appeared to be increasing, and hallucinogen (including 3, 4-methylenedioxymethamphetamine [MDMA] and lysergic acid diethylamide [LSD]), heroin, and sedative use, which appeared steady. Use of cocaine, amphetamine, and methamphetamine declined during the study period (Johnston et al. 2008).

Early Detection in Adolescents

Signs of adolescent drug use include a drop in school performance, irritability, apathy, mood change (including depression), poor self-care, weight loss, oversensitivity with regard to questions about drinking or drugs, and sudden changes in friends. Screening instruments targeted toward adolescents should be included in routine medical examinations before camp or in school. The use of urine analysis may help confirm a diagnosis when necessary. Early detection efforts are vital because it is increasingly recognized that a younger age at onset of addiction is associated with poorer outcomes, including alcohol-related harm, and a greater potential for clinically significant use (Bachman et al. 1991).

Contributing Factors

Peer group, school environment, age, geography, race, values, family attitudes toward substance abuse, risk-seeking temperament, and biological predisposition are all contributing factors to adolescent substance abuse. Nonuser adolescents are more likely than users to describe close relationships with their parents. Abstinent youth are more likely to be comfortably dependent on their parents and closer to family than users, who often describe themselves as independent and distant. Users more frequently indicate that they do not want to be like their parents and do not feel they need parental approval; they disclaim a desire for affection from their parents. Divorced children are at greater risk of substance abuse. Finally, an extensive literature focuses on the risks that come from being the victim of sexual abuse in childhood, and one twin study of more than 6,000 twins found an association between childhood sexual abuse and the later misuse of nicotine, alcohol, and other substances (Nelson et al. 2006).

Frequently, there is a positive family history for chemical dependence in adolescents with substance abuse problems. Genetic studies indicate a strong hereditary predisposition to alcoholism. If children do not abuse substances by age 21 years, they are unlikely to do so after that point.

Physical activity has been studied as a positive factor in reducing substance use in adolescents. At least for nicotine and cannabis, engagement in physical activity has been found to be inversely related to use.

In terms of tobacco, experimentation is common in adolescence; use is highly affected by environmental features (Brook et al. 2009). The risk that some smoking as an adolescent will lead to smoking as a young adult has an odds ratio of 16 (Chassin et al. 1996), but further research has reviewed the effects of peers, employment, education, and parental influences on the transition to young adult smoking. Greater physical activity is associated with reduced progression to significant use (Rodriguez and Audrain-McGovern 2004), and sports participation has been found to be protective, even among individuals who have the alleles seen as risk factors for smoking (Audrain-McGovern et al. 2006). At any point along the way, adolescents should be encouraged to refrain from first use and to stop if they have been experimenting with smoking tobacco.

Role of Families in Treatment

Families play a more important role in SUD treatment for adolescent relative to adult substance abusers. Parents and family members of adolescent abusers may be less resistant to involvement in treatment because the adolescent usually resides with them and they may feel responsible for the adolescent's behavior. When parents themselves are actively addicted, the challenges of treatment are greater. Adolescents are less likely than adults to enter treatment to avoid incarceration but are more likely than adults to be pushed into treatment—by their families, by schools, and/or by pediatricians and family physicians.

Residential Treatment

Inpatient or residential treatment for adolescents is indicated for those who have had a drug problem that has interfered with their ability to function in school, work, and home environments, and who have been unable to maintain abstinence through outpatient treatment. Low motivation for change, a disruptive home life, high acting-out, involvement with the juvenile justice system, and comorbid psychiatric or medical problems all may be reasons for inpatient treatment. Depression, suicidality, hyperactivity, chemical dependence, and drug overdoses are additional indications for residential treatment. Adolescents frequently require longer hospital stays than adults because of greater dispositional problems, more resistance to treatment, greater difficulty in controlling acting-out behavior during outpatient therapy, and greater severity of family problems. Treatment outcomes for adolescents are worse than those for adults. Predictors of treatment completion include greater severity of alcohol abuse; greater abuse of drugs other than alcohol, nicotine, or cannabis; higher degree of internalizing problems; and lower self-esteem (Blood and Cornwall 1994).

Substance Intoxication or Psychosis

Intoxication with drugs and alcohol in adolescents may lead to disinhibition, violence, and medical complications. Strategies for managing these crises include providing a quiet, supportive environment to minimize the chance of the child or adolescent acting out in a violent manner, and, if necessary, administering a benzodiazepine or atypical antipsychotic. Support staff may be needed to approach potentially violent adolescents and may have an additional quieting effect. Even in the absence of formally diagnosed comorbid conditions, use of substances among youth increases several risks, including getting into fights, carrying weapons, using other substances, and engaging in risky suicidal or sexual behaviors (DeWit et al. 2000). Police should be involved if the adolescent is carrying a weapon. Emergency room checks for weapons are very important when dealing with adolescents. Administration of sedatives should be avoided in adolescents who abuse substances, because benzodiazepines can cause disinhibition and increase the possibility of violent acting-out.

Mentally Ill, Chemically Abusing Adolescents

Although the risks vary by diagnosis, all childhood psychiatric disorders are associated with SUDs. Most adolescents entering inpatient drug and alcohol treatment programs have additional mental health problems, including conduct disorder, affective disorder, attention-deficit/hyperactivity disorder (ADHD), anxiety disorders, eating disorders, and other Axis I conditions, as well as frequent characterological diagnosis of passive-aggressive personality, borderline personality disorder, and narcissistic personality disorder. Conduct disorder is one of the strongest risk factors for early drinking, more so than ADHD itself (Moss and Lynch 2001). In terms of ADHD, repeated studies have demonstrated no additional risk of future substance use, depending on management with stimulant medications; in fact, the opposite has been shown (Biederman et al. 2006). The treatment of ADHD with methylphenidate in adolescents significantly reduces the risk of developing substance abuse in later life (Biederman et al. 1997).

Suicidal ideation and behavior is important in this population. Early initiation of alcohol use has been shown to be strongly associated with suicide attempts (Swahn et al. 2008). During assessment, careful history-taking regarding suicidal thoughts and suicide attempts is crucial. If there is a positive family history of suicide or depression, psychosis, isolation from families and friends, previous suicide attempts, clear-cut plans of suicide attempts, or violent means of carrying out the plan, the risk of suicide is increased. SUDs are major risk factors for suicide among adolescents.

Alcohol-related motor vehicle accidents are the leading cause of death among youth ages 15–24 years. There has also been a rash of recent reports of respiratory depression, coma, and death after excessive bouts of alcohol ingestion and after use of designer drugs such as MDMA (Ecstasy) (Schifano et al. 2006).

Increased alcohol and drug abuse in adolescents is frequently associated with risk-taking behavior linked to the spread of human immunodeficiency virus (HIV) infection (e.g., intravenous drug use, unsafe sexual practices, and increased sexual activity with multiple partners). Substance use disorders in adolescents may also directly and indirectly affect the immune system. Sexual abuse of children and adolescents is not uncommon in families with SUDs, and if the perpetrating family member is HIV positive, there is a further risk of spreading HIV infection.

Assessment

Assessment of the adolescent drug user must be comprehensive. It requires a careful history of both patient and family, including where and when drugs are used, the circumstances under which use occurs, the dosages used, and what drug effects and reactions have been experienced. Parents should be asked about the adolescent's behavior, personality changes, school performance and absenteeism, changes in peer affiliations, presence of rebelliousness, and number of occasions they thought their adolescent was intoxicated. Parental and sibling drug use history is also important. Parents' reactions to the adolescent's drug use, whether parents have confronted the adolescent about the drug use, and the adolescent's responses to such confrontation are important. Gathering histories from schools, pediatricians, clergy, and probation officers is also useful. The clinician should be aware of the possibility of denial by the adolescent or family.

Clinical Management Issues

The treatment of adolescents requires both structure and flexibility. Awareness of the possibility of contraband stashes and the necessity for intermittent urine screening is important in inpatient treatment programs to monitor compliance. Most programs rely heavily on a therapeutic milieu with individualized treatment planning. A warm, supportive environment with organized structure increases motivation and maximizes positive interaction with the peer group. Adolescent programs rely heavily on peer-support groups, family therapy, school, education on drug abuse, and 12-Step programs such as Alcoholics Anonymous (AA) and Alateen vocational programs, patient–staff meetings, and activity therapy. Programs that have the greatest success with adolescents encourage openness and spontaneous expression of feelings, allow patients to engage in independent decision making, have counselors help patients solve their real problems, use cognitive and behavioral approaches and relaxation techniques, have experienced counselors and staff, and frequently employ the support of volunteers. Cognitive-behavioral approaches have been modified for adolescents, and treatment manuals are available to help in the application of this efficacious modality.

Psychopharmacology

The increased focus on adolescent addiction has led to new approaches. When considering pharmacological interventions in children or adolescents, great care and attention are absolutely required. Disulfiram is rarely prescribed in adolescents. Withdrawal from alcohol is seldom a clinically significant syndrome in this population; when it occurs, however, it should be monitored and treated as it would be for adults. Bupropion, particularly in the sustained-release (SR) formulation at 150 mg/day, is safe and effective for adolescents who require assistance in smoking cessation (Muramoto et al. 2007). Finally, there is evidence that cognitive-behavioral therapy in combination with fluoxetine is superior to cognitive-behavioral therapy with placebo in the treatment of youths with depression and SUDs (Riggs et al. 2007).

Relapse Prevention

Relapse prevention is often more difficult with adolescents than with adults, and the goal of total abstinence is correspondingly harder to achieve. Rules that expel the patient after one instance of drug use ("one drug use and you're out") are less likely to be effective in adolescent treatment services, where youth may be all to eager to escape treatment. With adolescents, a slip needs to be understood as a symptom of the problem; the patient should not be rejected because of a relapse. Relapses may lead to adjustment of treatment plans and may require rehospitalization. Discharge planning must include outpatient treatment for drug abuse and frequent attendance at self-help support groups. Frequently, family or group treatments are added to individual treatment, depending on need. Urine screening for drug and alcohol is frequently part of a comprehensive outpatient plan. Adolescents may also need halfway houses, residential treatment centers, and, in some instances, long-term inpatient psychiatric care.

Primary, Secondary, and Tertiary Prevention

The addiction literature is focused on the mechanisms and risks of initiation, progression, and maintenance of use of abused substances among children and adolescents, highlighting the importance of applying primary, secondary, and tertiary prevention efforts to this population. Although identifying those at risk is an important first step, current methods of prevention in this population avoid stirring interest and curiosity and instead concentrate more on teaching "life skills" that support self-esteem, social skills, and assertiveness training (Botvin et al. 1995). A rule of thumb for all adolescent populations and all substances is that prevention of initiation is beneficial, and any delays in initiation have a beneficial effect in reducing progression—the longer that adolescents postpone initiation, the better (Hingson et al. 2006).

Educational Programs

Primary prevention efforts have focused heavily on school-based and work-based alcohol education programs and mass media campaigns, as well as attempts to limit availability of the agent. Programs targeted toward students, parents, and employees have significantly increased knowledge regarding alcohol and drug abuse. It is harder to achieve changes in attitudes toward alcohol and drugs, and changes in drinking behavior have been modest or difficult to demonstrate.

Efforts at life-skills training focusing on values clarification abilities, decision making, and drug refusal may be more effective in changing attitudes than cognitive interventions aimed at increasing knowledge alone. Programs (based on social learning theory) that teach young people how to refuse drugs provide information about the hazards of drugs, peer pressure, and means of expanding specific behavioral repertoires for saying no. Through rehearsal of a variety of rejecting responses, it is hoped that in the appropriate situation, these responses will be available. These programs often begin in middle school (usually from sixth to ninth grade) and use peer leaders to enhance social resistance skills through improved self-management and self-efficacy. Factors that increase adolescent substance abuse include peer pressure, negative role models, desire to attain adult status, curiosity, low self-esteem, and family instability. Drugs may be used to numb painful affects, initiate sexual intimacy, and promote greater group identification. Student assistance model programs include 1) education and groups, with children of alcoholics especially targeted; 2) treatment or referral for substance-abusing students; 3) early screening of students who manifest behavioral changes; and 4) work with parents and community groups.

Adolescents frequently experiment with alcohol and drug use. A national program of teaching children to refuse substances has been successful only in part. Because of the ubiquitous presence of alcohol in our culture, coming to personal terms with alcohol and drug abuse may represent a developmental task for some teenagers. A "just say no" approach may be most important for those at highest risk for developing an alcohol problem, such as children of alcoholics. In addition, adolescents need to be educated on what the reasons for saying no are in the first place. Most educational programs touch on myths about alcohol, alcohol advertisement, causes of alcoholism, and the effects of alcohol and drugs on life satisfaction, and also instill positive social skills and behaviors.

Twelve-Step and Other Self-Help Programs

Self-help groups such as Alateen, Al-Anon, AA, and Adult Children of Alcoholics provide support and disseminate educational materials. Groups such as Mothers Against Drunk Driving exert important lobbying power. These organizations also help disseminate information and, indirectly through 12-Step work, aid in early case-finding and intervention.

Neurodevelopmental Effects of Maternal Substance Use on the Fetus

In addition to extensive data on fetal alcohol syndrome and fetal alcohol spectrum disorder, the literature contains a variety of studies and information about the residual effects of maternal substance use during gestation. In all of these cases, the best evidence has controlled for factors other than the substance use, but in real-world cases, the non–substance use issues may pose risks to the fetus that are as great as, if not greater than, the risks posed by the substance use itself. Alcohol and tobacco are the two substances for which the most substantial and serious long-term neurodevelopment risks have been discerned, but it must be maintained that any substance use during pregnancy imposes medical and neurological/neurodevelopmental risks to the fetus and the mother and to the success of the pregnancy overall. Any use should be followed by extensive evaluation and assessment.

Alcohol

Fetal alcohol syndrome incidence is approximately 1–3 per 1,000 live births generally and as high as 1 in 100 births in some Eskimo villages (Stratton et al. 1996). Typical signs of fetal alcohol syndrome include low birth weight, growth deficiency with delayed motor development, mental retardation and learning problems, and other less severe fetal alcohol behavioral effects. No safe alcohol level during pregnancy has been established, and dangers increase with amounts used. Fetal alcohol spectrum disorder (FASD) is a term that reflects acceptance that a broader group of effects may be present below the threshold for the full fetal alcohol syndrome.

Cocaine and Stimulants

For live births, the risk of serious congenital malformations or medical complications from prenatal cocaine exposure has been found to be minimal, but other morbidities have been shown to follow exposure. In terms of outcome studies, placement in school special education programs has been found to follow prenatal cocaine use (Levine et al. 2008). The effects of prenatal cocaine exposure on intelligence are more subtle than originally thought, and problematic behavioral conditions have been inconsistently documented. Aside from intelligence, there are findings that a variety of cognitive functions are often affected, but not in a manner that is predictable.

Tobacco

An active literature documents the neurodevelopmental effects of exposure to tobacco or nicotine during gestation. In addition to increased risk of placenta previa, placental abruption, placental infarcts, and placental changes due to vasoconstriction, maternal smoking during pregnancy is associated with increased risk of sudden infant death syndrome and other deaths up to age 5 years in the exposed child. In terms of behavioral issues, however, smoking during pregnancy has been associated with toddler negativity (Brook et al. 2000), externalizing behavior problems, internalizing behavior (Orlebeke et al. 1997), aggression conduct disorder (Wakschlag and Hans 2002), oppositional defiant behavior, criminal behavior, and psychiatric morbidity (Cornelius et al. 2001).

Postnatal tobacco exposure is significant as well. Reports have supported an association between behavior abnormalities and postnatal tobacco exposure. Impulsivity at age 10 years may be more affected by postnatal than prenatal exposure. One study has reported a higher rate of externalizing behavior problems in 5-year-old children with both prenatal and postnatal tobacco exposures than with prenatal exposure only (Eskenazi and Castorina 1999).

Cannabis

After adjustment for other factors, some studies have found no replicable syndromal effects due to prenatal marijuana exposure. However, other investigations found significant associations between prenatal marijuana exposure and hyperactivity, impulsivity, inattention, delinquency, and externalizing behavior (Goldschmidt et al. 2000).

Opioids

Studies have demonstrated a prenatal opiate exposure effect on externalizing behavior problems only at age 5 years. This is separate from the issue of potential intoxication and withdrawal at the neonatal period. No pregnant woman should ever receive naloxone (e.g., Narcan), and clonidine should be avoided. In neonatal abstinence syndrome, the infant's capacity to breast-feed may be impaired, and other serious effects, such as seizures, are not infrequent (see Chapter 6, "Natural Histories of Substance Abuse"). If given without naloxone, buprenorphine is a safe medication during pregnancy; however, when mixed with naloxone, it poses risks. Although buprenorphine is expressed in breast milk, it has poor oral bioavailability, so it is relatively better than the presence of other opioids in breast milk. Abstinence syndromes should be suspected and assessed in infants who will not breast-feed.

Key Points

- Any postponement or delay in initiation of use of substances of abuse among adolescents provides lower risk of future progression of use.

- Substance abuse in teens is associated with disinhibited behavior, violence, suicide, and comorbid Axis I disorders.
- Effective treatments include inpatient and residential treatment, behavioral approaches, and pharmacological interventions.
- Substance abuse by pregnant women can lead to negative outcomes of the pregnancy, both in the short-term as well as in the long-term development of the child after birth.
- Any prenatal substance use raises medical, obstetric, pediatric, and psychosocial risks.

References

American Academy of Child and Adolescent Psychiatry: Practice parameters for the assessment and treatment of children and adolescents with substance use disorders. J Am Acad Child Adolesc Psychiatry 36:140S–156S, 1997

Audrain-McGovern J, Rodriguez D, Wileyto EP, et al: Effect of team sport participation on genetic predisposition to adolescent smoking progression. Arch Gen Psychiatry 63:433–441, 2006

Bachman JG, Wallace JM Jr, O'Malley PM: Racial/ethnic differences in smoking, drinking, and illicit drug use among American high school seniors, 1976–1989. Am J Public Health 81:372–377, 1991

Biederman J, Wilens T, Mick E, et al: Is ADHD a risk factor for psychoactive substance use disorders? Findings from a four-year prospective follow-up study. J Am Acad Child Adolesc Psychiatry 36:21–29, 1997

Biederman J, Monuteaux MC, Mick E, et al: Is cigarette smoking a gateway to alcohol and illicit drug use disorders? A study of youths with and without attention deficit hyperactivity disorder. Biol Psychiatry 59:258–264, 2006

Blood L, Cornwall A: Pretreatment variables that predict completion of an adolescent substance abuse treatment program. J Nerv Ment Dis 182:14–19, 1994

Botvin GJ, Baker E, Dusenbury L, et al: Long-term follow-up results of a randomized drug abuse prevention trial in a white middle-class population. JAMA 273:1106–12, 1995

Brook JS, Brook DW, Whiteman M: The influence of maternal smoking during pregnancy on the toddler's negativity. Arch Pediatr Adolesc Med 154:381–385, 2000

Brook JS, Saar NS, Zhang C, et al: Familial and non-familial smoking: effects on smoking and nicotine dependence. Drug Alcohol Depend 101:62–68, 2009

Chassin L, Presson CC, Rose JS, et al: The natural history of cigarette smoking from adolescence to adulthood: demographic predictors of continuity and change. Health Psychol 15:478–484, 1996

Cornelius MD, Ryan CM, Day NL, et al: Prenatal tobacco effects on neuropsychological outcomes among preadolescents. J Dev Behav Pediatr 22:217–225, 2001

DeWit DJ, Adlaf EM, Offord DR, et al: Age at first alcohol use: a risk factor for the development of alcohol disorders. Am J Psychiatry 157:745–750, 2000

Eskenazi B, Castorina R: Association of prenatal maternal or postnatal child environmental tobacco smoke exposure and neurodevelopmental and behavioral problems in children. Environ Health Perspect 107:991–1000, 1999

Goldschmidt L, Day NL, Richardson GA: Effects of prenatal marijuana exposure on child behavior problems at age 10. Neurotoxicol Teratol 22:325–336, 2000

Hingson RW, Heeren T, Winter MR: Age at drinking onset and alcohol dependence: age at onset, duration, and severity. Arch Pediatr Adolesc Med 160:739–746, 2006

Johnston LD, O'Malley PM, Bachman JG, et al: Various stimulant drugs show continuing gradual declines among teens in 2008, most illicit drugs hold steady. Ann Arbor, MI, University of Michigan News Service, December 11, 2008. Available at: http://www.monitoringthefuture.org. Accessed February 22, 2009.

Levine TP, Liu J, Das A, et al: Effects of prenatal cocaine exposure on special education. Pediatrics 122:e83–e91, 2008

Moss H, Lynch KG: Comorbid disruptive behavior disorder symptoms and their relationship to adolescent alcohol use disorders. Drug Alcohol Depend 64:75–83, 2001

Muramoto ML, Leischow SJ, Sherrill D, et al: Randomized, double-blind, placebo-controlled trial of 2 dosages of sustained-release bupropion for adolescent smoking cessation. Arch Pediatr Adolesc Med 161:1068–1074, 2007

Nelson EC, Heath AC, Lynskey MT, et al: Childhood sexual abuse and risks for licit and illicit drug-related outcomes: a twin study. Psychol Med 36:1473–1483, 2006

Orlebeke JF, Knol DL, Verhulst FC: Increase in child behavior problems resulting from maternal smoking during pregnancy. Arch Environ Health 52:317–321, 1997

Riggs PD, Mikulich-Gilbertson SK, Davies RD, et al: A randomized controlled trial of fluoxetine and cognitive behavioral therapy in adolescents with major depression, behavior problems, and substance use disorders. Arch Pediatr Adolesc Med 161:1026–1034, 2007

Rodriguez D, Audrain-McGovern J: Team sport participation and smoking: analysis with general growth mixture modeling. J Pediatric Psychology 29:299–308, 2004

Schifano F, Corkery J, Deluca P, et al: Ecstasy (MDMA, MDA, MDEA, MBDB) consumption, seizures, related offences, prices, dosage levels and deaths in the UK (1994–2003). J Psychopharmacol 20:456–463, 2006

Stratton KR, Howe CJ, Battaglia FC, et al: Fetal Alcohol Syndrome: Research Base for Diagnostic Criteria, Epidemiology, Prevention, and Treatment. Institute of Medicine, Division of Biobehavioral Sciences and Mental Disorders, Committee to Study Fetal Alcohol Syndrome, National Institute on Alcohol Abuse and Alcoholism. Washington, DC, National Academies Press, 1996

Swahn MH, Bossarte RM, Sullivent EE 3rd, et al: Age of alcohol use initiation, suicidal behavior, and peer and dating violence victimization and perpetration among high-risk, seventh-grade adolescents. Pediatrics 121:297–305, 2008

Wakschlag LS, Hans SL: Maternal smoking during pregnancy and conduct problems in high-risk youth: a developmental framework. Dev Psychopathol 14:351–369, 2002

10

Specific Populations

This chapter covers issues specific to several clinical populations, groups in which substance use is associated with particular patterns, effects, or epidemiological aspects: women, the elderly, chronically disabled or homeless individuals, and others.

Women

There are several differences between men and women regarding the use of substances and their effects. Low doses of alcohol have greater effects on women than on men, and although no more than 2 drinks per day may be healthy for men, for women the equivalent is 1. In the United States, the male:female ratio of alcoholism is 3:1. However, the ratio is generally 1:1 for all other substances except for prescription drugs, which are disproportionately used by women (Warner et al. 1995). Women are underrepresented in treatment programs, and their special needs are often not addressed during treatment. Yet the stigma of substance use disorders (SUDs) affects women gravely. Women suffer greater medical morbidity secondary to addictions

than do men (Ashley et al. 1977). Traditionally, women with SUDs are identified differently from men. Whereas violence or other reckless behavior often
brings men with SUDs to clinical attention, women abusers mostly reach
treatment through nonviolent scenarios, such as employee assistance programs, family interventions, or obstetric/gynecological evaluations. (However,
some data show that more substance-abusing women are violent than was previously thought [Eronen 1995].) The potential for fetal alcohol syndrome and
human immunodeficiency virus (HIV) transmission contribute greater ur-
gency to identification of female alcoholism and intravenous drug use.
Women more frequently present with coexisting panic, anxiety, mood, and
eating disorders compared with men, and women less frequently have accom-
panying antisocial problems. Women who experienced sexual abuse as children often develop alcoholism and drug abuse as adults. Women suffer greatly
from and are profoundly affected by the abuse of fathers and husbands with
alcoholism. Women who abuse alcohol have a later onset and a more rapid
progression of substance abuse and consume a smaller amount of alcohol relative to male alcoholics. They are also more likely than men to have a significant other who is also a substance abuser, and women who abuse alcohol have
higher rates of comorbid psychiatric disorders.

Women with alcohol SUDs are also more likely than men to attempt suicide and less likely to complete it. They also tend to have a history of sexual or
physical abuse and to date the onset of the SUD to a stressful event. Women
with alcohol SUDs have a higher mortality rate and are more likely to report
previous psychiatric treatment than are men. Women with cocaine SUDs have
a more rapid progression of the disease, use less often than men with cocaine
SUDs, usually have a spouse who also has an SUD, and have a greater likelihood of suicide attempts than men. On the other hand, among female cocaine
users there are fewer transitions between sobriety and use (Gallop et al. 2007).

Genetic, Cultural, and Biological Effects

Most research on the heredity of alcoholism has been done with men. Recent
studies indicate that a genetic potential for alcoholism exists in women as well,
although it may very well be that this is frequently overridden by cultural
norms. Alcoholism in women varies markedly, depending on the culture. For
Koreans, the male:female ratio for alcoholism is 1:28. Women have a higher

blood alcohol level (BAL) pound-per-pound per drink compared with men, and their BALs vary over the course of the menstrual cycle. Women are most frequently admitted to alcohol treatment hospitals during the perimenstrual stage, which is often marked by heavier drinking. In addition to a lower tolerance for alcohol, women tend to have a more telescoped course of the chronic effects of excessive drinking, including cirrhosis of the liver, compared with men. These gender differences may be partially explained by the fact that men have greater amounts of alcohol dehydrogenase in the gastric mucosa. Alcohol and drugs in women may initially be used to reduce sexual inhibitions; however, alcohol ultimately reduces desire and ability to perform sexually in women, as in men, and recovery usually leads to better sexual function.

Psychiatric Comorbidity

Women with SUDs more often have mood disorders than do men. In fact, with the exception of attention-deficit disorder (ADD) and antisocial personality disorder, women have a greater prevalence of comorbid psychopathology, particularly anxiety disorders (especially posttraumatic stress disorder) and eating disorders (Kessler et al. 1995). Secondary alcoholism with self-medication for anxiety or depression is much more frequent in women than in men. Sometimes, alcoholism may develop after benzodiazepine dependence, which may have started during efforts to treat anxiety disorders.

Treatment Issues

Women in traditional treatment programs often experience discomfort when talking about sexual abuse and sexual issues in mixed male–female groups. Women may feel intimidated and outnumbered by men in alcohol rehabilitation programs. Thus, women's groups and special programs and residences for women in rehabilitation programs are beneficial. In general, although treatment for alcoholism and drug abuse in women is similar in many ways to that in men, tailoring of the treatment is needed to address gender differences. Special treatment considerations include watching especially closely for the possibility of sedative-hypnotic dependence, anxiety disorders, depression, extrasensitivity to stigma, dealing with abusive spouses, and awareness of fetal alcohol and drug effects. Contact with recovered alcoholic women role models and working with female professionals may also be a factor in improved self-esteem.

Evidence of differences between men and women in their response to psychosocial therapies for substance use disorders is growing. Awareness of the possibility that addicted women may be associated with addicted or abusive male partners must be present at all times, and this must be taken into account when making treatment plans for women. Utilization of couples therapies should be considered (see Chapter 12, "Treatment Modalities") (Fals-Stewart et al. 2006).

The care of women of childbearing age with SUDs requires a great deal of attention. Careful use of medication in women of childbearing age includes awareness of relative risks and benefits. Treatment of depression and anxiety disorders in women with dual diagnosis is often necessary. Inpatient treatment poses special problems for young mothers, and few programs exist in which women can be hospitalized along with their children. Alcoholic women have greater fears of loss of custody and increased needs for child-care services. Women frequently have economic problems that may make it more difficult for them to get good treatment. Although alcoholic men are frequently married to nonalcoholic women who are supportive of their husbands' recovery, more often women with alcoholism are married to addicted men who may be less helpful or even harmful toward recovery. Women may need to separate from an addicted, abusing spouse to get well, and often need help for sobriety from sober women friends and female role models who are in the process of recovery. General aspects of the care of addicted women are presented in Table 10–1 (Blume 2005).

Women who smoke tobacco and become pregnant are faced with the need to quit rapidly, especially when the pregnancy is a surprise. The capacity to quit, if at least temporarily, during gestation in this population tends to be high (McBride et al. 1999). Women's capacity to quit addictions in general may be enhanced by the experience of pregnancy and the motivation to stay healthy for the sake of a fetus or a child (see Chapter 9, "Children and Adolescents," for a review of the effects of prenatal and postnatal exposure of infants to tobacco).

Table 10–1. Special considerations in treatment of women

Psychiatric assessment for comorbid disorders; date of onset for each (primary/ secondary)

Attention to past history and present risk of physical and sexual assault

Assessment of prescription drug abuse/dependence

Comprehensive physical examination for physical complications and comorbid disorders

Need for access to health care (including obstetric care)

Psychoeducation to include information on substance use in pregnancy

Child-care services for women in treatment

Parenting education and assistance

Evaluation and treatment of significant others and children

Positive female role models (among treatment staff, friends, self-help)

Attention to guilt, shame, and self-esteem issues

Assessment and treatment of sexual dysfunction

Attention to the effects of sexism in the previous experience of the patient (e.g., underemployment, lack of opportunity, rigid sex roles)

Avoidance of iatrogenic drug dependence

Special attention to the needs of minority women, lesbian women, and those in the criminal justice system

Source. Blume 2005.

Problems Secondary to Addiction in Women

General Medical Conditions

Women who abuse substances are at risk of developing a number of specific general medical conditions, and, compared with men, when they develop such secondary conditions, they occur at a faster rate and with higher morbidity, a phenomenon known as "telescoping." Alcoholic cardiomyopathy and cirrhosis occur at a faster rate in women than in men (Urbano-Marquez et al. 1995). Studies have shown that women who abuse alcohol are at greater risk of developing breast cancer than are nondrinking women (Longnecker et al. 1988). Female SUD patients require comprehensive follow-up in the primary care setting.

Acquired Immunodeficiency Syndrome

The spread of HIV has produced a growing pandemic whose effects are seen every day among women with SUDs, especially minority women. A majority of women in methadone programs in urban centers are HIV positive; a majority of these women are also mothers. Female prostitution can be another cause of the spread of acquired immunodeficiency syndrome (AIDS) and is also frequently associated with intravenous drug use.

A special concern of women is the possibility of contracting AIDS through intercourse with HIV-positive men who are intravenous drug users or bisexual. Women who abuse substances may frequently take more risks, have poorer self-care, and less frequently insist on safe sex. Women of childbearing age who are intravenous users are at especially high risk and need careful counseling.

Effects on Sexual and Reproductive Function

Sexual function is affected by almost all drugs of abuse. Despite its reputation, alcohol is not an aphrodisiac, and all sexually active female alcoholics should be reminded that sexual function improves with sobriety (Gavaler et al. 1995). Libido is decreased as a result of cocaine and amphetamine use. Also, heroin disrupts ovulation. It should be noted that the treatment of neonates for methadone withdrawal is a common procedure, and methadone use is not an absolute contraindication to pregnancy (Brown et al. 1998). Cocaine can cause placental abruption and ventricular tachycardia in the neonate (Volpe 1992).

The Elderly

The true scope of alcohol and drug abuse problems in the geriatric population is unknown. The incidence of alcoholism is lower in the elderly population. A greater and more frequent problem is overuse of prescription drugs and interaction of alcohol and other medications being used. Diagnosis is often more difficult in the elderly; denial of problems is frequent. Age-related changes in the pharmacokinetics of drugs with enhanced sensitivity to drugs and use of multiple drugs contribute to more severe consequences of substance abuse in the elderly. Substance abuse in the elderly may have late onset as a reaction to the stresses of advanced age, including retirement, loss of spouse and friends, and problems with health. Chronic heavy alcohol and substance abuse often lead to premature death, which may in part account for reduction of incidence of chronic alcoholism in the elderly. In addition to selective survival, it has also been postulated that cohort differences contribute to various patterns of cultural acceptance of substance use in different generations. This hypothesis would be consistent with future increases in geriatric alcoholism. It is essential to keep in mind at all times that elderly alcoholics (especially males) are at very high risk of suicide.

Special Problems in Diagnosis

Alcoholism is less likely to be detected in retired people because impairments in social and occupational functioning may not be obvious. Elderly alcoholics frequently have fewer antisocial problems, and it may be difficult to distinguish the consequences of substance use from aging itself. Cognitive problems are frequent in the elderly in general. Even though they are accelerated by alcoholism, cognitive problems may be wrongly attributed to degenerative brain disease. The hazards of heavy alcohol use on sleep, sexual functioning, and cognitive ability potentiate the changes that ordinarily occur with aging and with the use of multiple medications.

Complications

The pharmacokinetic changes that normally accompany aging include a relatively increased volume of distribution, greater central nervous system sensitivity to toxic substances, and metabolic changes, including a diminished capacity of the liver to carry out primary enzymatic degradation. The common polypharmacy of the elderly contributes to this problem. Alcohol's liver effects potentiate the possibility of overdose and with some drugs may lead to a more rapid metabolism, which may affect the clinical effectiveness of medications needed by the elderly. Alcohol's depressant effects may further contribute to major depression and cognitive impairment. Some elderly patients experience a loss of tolerance to alcohol, which leads to more intense effects with relatively small doses. The dementia that results from alcoholism is not reversible but does not progress upon cessation of drinking (Saunders et al. 1991). Thiamine deficiency is a common etiology of dementia in elderly alcoholics, and in those cases repletion should be instituted in a timely fashion lest it progress to Wernicke's encephalopathy.

Table 10–2.   Guidelines in caring for the elderly

Avoid use of disulfiram.

Use short-acting benzodiazepines.

Realize that older patients may be less likely to achieve full abstinence.

Consider each patient's life experiences.

Institute thiamine repletion when needed.

Treatment Issues

Greater creativity, flexibility, and sensitivity is required to address the needs of elderly individuals. Geriatric patients may need to be protected from threatening and acting-out behaviors of younger patients. Elderly patients also require somewhat less confrontation, a greater degree of support, and more attention to work with family members. The consequences of divorce are likely to also be greater in this group, and spouses are less likely to do well if left because of a drinking problem. Table 10–2 offers general guidelines for treating elderly individuals with alcoholism.

Prescription Drug Abuse

Abuse of prescription drugs is a common problem in the elderly (Abrams and Alexopoulos 1988). Polypharmacy and sensitivity to toxic effects frequently lead elderly patients into difficulty. Not infrequently, stopping medications may cause an apparent dementia to resolve. Benzodiazepine abuse among women is common, and sleep medications contribute to the problem. Memory problems may lead to unintentional misuse and overuse of prescription drugs. Inadequate explanation of the way medication should be taken and misunderstanding of dosage instructions are other problems that occur. Ambulatory abusers of these medications may require hospitalization in order to discontinue use. Nursing home patients are sometimes overmedicated to control disruptiveness and to reduce demands on nursing staff.

Chronic, Disabled, and Homeless Patients

Chronic psychoactive substance–dependent patients are a group with polysubstance abuse involving a wide range of substances, extensive and varied experience with treatment, and vast demographic disparities. A common feature of this group is maladaptive use of drugs of abuse over a long period of time (at least 1 year) with recurrent disability in physical, social, academic, or vocational functioning. This population is frequently in need of long-term institutional treatment, and there is a paucity of resources available for sophisticated, targeted treatment of the multiple challenges these patients often face. The effectiveness of specific treatments and combinations of treatments has not been clearly established, and the problems posed by this population are serious. Unfortunately, Veterans Administration hospitals have reduced the availability of inpatient care to veterans, which affects many elderly persons with SUDs.

The chronic patient may be severely stigmatized, possibly because his or her condition is seen as self-inflicted. However, unlike other maladaptive behavior, such as cigarette smoking (leading to emphysema) or lack of compliance with a low-salt diet (contributing to congestive heart failure), the self-inflicted aspect of addiction has led to prejudice in regard to allocation of resources and handling of benefits and disability. Chronic psychoactive substance–dependent patients may need a wide range of services and links with other programs in the community. Programs must be culturally relevant and meet local realities of communities. Highly trained staffs with positive attitudes about treatment are needed for implementing treatment of patients with multiple problems.

Cognitively Impaired Patients With Chronic Substance Dependence

The cognitive impairment that is associated with chronic alcohol and drug dependence is likely to affect the ability of patients to handle cognitive treatment programs. In addition, patients with Korsakoff's syndrome, alcohol dementia, and other severe complications of alcoholism and drug abuse may be in need of chronic nursing home care. Many treatment failures in alcohol and drug treatment programs are based on unappreciated difficulties that patients have in processing information.

Patients With Chronic Mental Illness and Substance Abuse

Chronic mental illness frequently contributes to the chronicity and severity of substance abuse problems. Facilities that combine psychiatric treatment with substance abuse rehabilitation techniques are often not available to these patients. Severely disturbed drug abusers may be shunned by drug rehabilitation facilities not equipped to handle them. Confrontational methods and overemphasis on a drug-free model, which in some facilities includes underprescribing of psychotropic medication, can be detrimental to the mentally ill.

Chronic Substance Abuse in the Multiply Disabled and Physically Handicapped

Alcohol and drug abuse may contribute to the development of another physical disability, such as paraplegia or head trauma. The physically disabled patient may have easier access to prescription drugs, and physicians may too readily prescribe medication out of a sense of guilt or futility. Disabled individuals who feel frustrated by and angry at being dependent, socially isolated, and discriminated against by the rest of society may be more vulnerable to depression, anxiety, self-hatred, low motivation, and low self-esteem. They are more likely to suffer from chronic pain, which may lead to iatrogenic addiction.

Blind and Deaf Patients With Substance Abuse

Blind and visually impaired patients may have problems coping with their impairment, which may contribute to substance abuse. Deaf patients may have greater denial of the existence of substance abuse problems within their community, are afraid of stigmatization in having an additional problem, and have a lack of adequate signs in sign language to symbolize drunkenness or sobriety. Innovative treatment programs using simultaneous translators in groups to mainstream deaf patients through alcohol rehabilitation programs have been tried. Unfortunately, there are few alcohol and drug counselors who are well trained in signing and not enough translators who can facilitate communication with such patients.

Substance-Abusing Patients With Spinal Cord Injury

The problems of alcohol and drug abuse in patients with spinal cord damage are significant. The spinal cord damage may have been caused by alcohol and substance abuse in the first place. Physical problems such as decubitus ulcers are caused by immobility and poor nutrition, which may be worsened by substance abuse. Treatment programs for alcoholic patients with spinal cord injury must be geared to offer a range of interventions, including physical rehabilitation, group psychotherapy, and 12-Step recovery groups such as Alcoholics Anonymous (AA) and Narcotics Anonymous (NA).

Intellectually Disabled Substance Users

Patients with mild intellectual disability (IQ of 55–70 and low adaptive functioning) think concretely, are easily manipulated, and may have problems learning from experience. Most of these patients live in the community and may attempt to socialize in neighborhood bars viewed as warm and nonjudgmental. Intellectually disabled patients may have a wish to feel accepted as part of a group, and alcohol and substance abuse are seen as a means of improving socialization. Treatment and prevention efforts must take into account the special needs of this population. Poor verbal skills may make it more difficult for mildly intellectually disabled individuals to benefit from AA and NA meetings and group programs that involve cognitive approaches and education about drug abuse. An emphasis on provision of a high degree of acceptance, warmth, and emotional support is needed in working with these patients. If mildly intellectually disabled patients are able to learn that they cannot drink safely and if simple messages of not drinking are reinforced, then they may do very well in treatment.

Homeless Patients With Addictions

Evidence shows that the homeless population is no longer principally composed of skid row alcoholics or single, older, chronic alcoholic men (Koegel and Burnam 1988). The population is getting younger and includes an increasing number of women; as many as 90% have a primary psychiatric diagnosis. In several different urban samples in the United States, 20%–60% of homeless patients reported alcohol dependence. These patients frequently do not receive welfare; are disconnected from a social network, including families; and are unable to use available social services. They often enter treatment through intervention by church groups, 12-Step programs, and posthospitalization detoxification. Clinics that work with homeless substance abusers struggle to obtain basic social support services with adequate provision for meals and a place to live. Many homeless individuals become entangled with law enforcement over charges that arise as they do things to survive (e.g., loitering, trespassing, aggressive panhandling), and the justice system's use of diversion techniques (e.g., mental health court) for these cases is important (Council of State Governments 2001).

Minority Populations

Alcohol and drug abuse is a major problem in subsets of minority populations (Franklin 2005). SUDs have had a major impact on overall life expectancies in blacks, Hispanics, and American Indians. Although, compared with whites, blacks have comparable rates of heavy drinking, blacks have suffered a disproportionate number of medical, psychological, and social sequelae. Blacks have twice the rate of cirrhosis and 10 times the rate of esophageal cancer in the 35- to 44-year age group. Hypertension is also a greater problem for black patients. Half of black homicide cases are alcohol related. The rates of substance abuse may be skewed somewhat due to statistics that rely heavily on public facilities. Blacks and Hispanics make up 12% and 7%, respectively, of the U.S. population but account for 26% and 14%, respectively, of the population with AIDS. Excessive alcohol consumption is also reported among rural and urban American Indians.

Targeting Treatment

Several researchers have been working in the area of minority substance abuse; however, there has been a paucity of information and data vitally needed in this area. We cannot assume that research and program design applicable to middle-class white Americans will be equally applicable to minority communities. There is a recognition of the need for culturally sensitive treatment programs in minority communities. The meaning of *culturally sensitive* is open to research and discussion. There are some culturally specific etiological and treatment-related problems. Unemployment, racism, poor self-esteem, corruption of cultural values, and economic exploitation are prevailing problems in urban black communities and may contribute to the high rates of psychoactive substance abuse. Blacks are more readily diagnosed with alcoholism than are whites and are often misdiagnosed psychiatrically. As teenagers, black individuals report less alcohol abuse than white teenagers; however, they quickly catch up and have comparable rates of abuse in their 20s and 30s. Although the biopsychosocial approach is equally valid in minorities, social factors such as poor education, unemployment, low job skills, racism, and substance-abusing peer role models become important etiological factors and must be addressed in any culturally sensitive program. Recognition and cooperation of indigenous cultural institutions such as churches are needed. Blacks have had less access to treatment in the past; cutbacks in funding of social agencies may further block access to treatment. Family treatment approaches are especially valuable in the Hispanic community. The importance of respect for cultural diversity is essential in drug treatment programs.

Cultural Patterns

Some observers have described a "sea change" in the American Indian community's increased concern over substance use among its members, although the excess use has persisted (Novins et al. 2000). American Indian culture includes the social tradition of the "drinking party," in which alcohol is consumed to excess and disinhibition is sanctioned. In Hispanic culture, there is the notion of machismo where manhood is equated with the ability to hold one's liquor. If a man is able to provide for his family, alcoholism may well be tolerated. Alcohol is often seen as a celebration of life and integrally related to holidays and festivals. Exposure of alcoholism often brings shame to the family and the community.

Treatment in minority communities generally must focus more on the extended family. Treatment programs and AA meetings must have some flexibility and respond to cultural norms. We must also recognize the heterogeneity within minority communities. For example, rural southern American black individuals may have different cultural norms compared with West Indian black individuals. In addition, minority women may have different roles and special treatment issues that are not prevalent in the majority population. In family therapy with Hispanic groups (e.g., families), attention to issues related to respect and machismo can lead to good results. There are unmet needs in American Indians with substance abuse problems, and we must address why that is and fix it (Gilder et al. 2008).

In summary, treatment personnel are faced with combining good basic alcohol and drug abuse treatment with cultural sensitivity and cultural competence. In reality, alcohol and drugs are going to remain a major problem within minority communities until we adequately address basic social ills.

Key Points

• Special populations pose specific treatment needs.
• Women, in particular, should be assessed for exposure to domestic violence or substance use by spouse.
• Some ethnic groups have specific biological, psychological, or social responses to substances of abuse.

References

Abrams RC, Alexopoulos GS: Alcohol and drug abuse: substance abuse in the elderly: over the counter and illegal drugs. Hosp Community Psychiatry 39:822–823, 1988

Ashley MJ, Olin JS, LeRiche WH, et al: Morbidity in alcoholics: evidence for accelerated development of physical disease in women. Arch Intern Med 137:883–887, 1977

Blume S: Addictive disorders in women, in Clinical Textbook of Addictive Disorders, 3rd Edition. Edited by Frances RJ, Miller SI, Mack AH. New York, Guilford, 2005, pp 437–456

Brown HL, Britton KA, Mahaffey D, et al: Methadone maintenance in pregnancy: a reappraisal. Am J Obstet Gynecol 179:459–463, 1998 ·

Council of State Governments: Criminal Justice/Mental Health Consensus Project. New York, Council of State Governments Justice Center, 2001

Eronen M: Mental disorders and homicidal behavior in female subjects. Am J Psychiatry 152:1216–1212, 1995

Fals-Stewart W, Birchler GR, Kelley ML: Learning sobriety together: a randomized clinical trial examining behavioral couples therapy with alcoholic female patients. J Consult Clin Psychol 74:579–591, 2006

Franklin J: Minority populations, in Clinical Textbook of Addictive Disorders, 3rd Edition. Edited by Frances RJ, Miller SI, Mack AH. New York, Guilford, 2005, pp 321–339

Gallop RJ, Crits-Christoph P, Ten Have TR, et al: Differential transitions between cocaine use and abstinence for men and women. J Consult Clin Psychol 75:95–103, 2007

Gavaler JS, Rizzo A, Rossaro L, et al: Sexuality of alcoholic women with menstrual cycle function: effects of duration of alcohol abstinence. Alcohol Clin Exp Res 17:778–781, 1995

Gilder DA, Lau P, Corey L, et al: Factors associated with remission from alcohol dependence in an American Indian community group. Am J Psychiatry 165:1172–1178, 2008

Kessler RC, Sonnega A, Bromet E, et al: Post-traumatic stress disorder in the national comorbidity survey. Arch Gen Psychiatry 52:1048–1060, 1995

Koegel P, Burnam A: Alcoholism among homeless adults in the inner city of Los Angeles. Arch Gen Psychiatry 45:1011–1018, 1988

Longnecker MP, Berlin JA, Orza MJ, et al: A meta-analysis of alcohol consumption in relation to breast cancer. JAMA 260:652–656, 1988

McBride CM, Curry SJ, Lando HA, et al: Prevention of relapse in women who quit smoking during pregnancy. Am J Public Health 89:706–711, 1999

Novins DK, Beals J, Sack WH, et al: Unmet needs for substance abuse and mental health services among northern plains American Indian adolescents. Psychiatric Services 51:1045–1047, 2000

Saunders PA, Copeland JRM, Dewey ME, et al: Heavy drinking as a risk factor for depression and dementia in elderly men. Br J Psychiatry 159:213–216, 1991

Urbano-Marquez A, Ramon E, Fernandez-Sola J, et al: The greater risk of alcoholic cardiomyopathy and myopathy in women compared with men. JAMA 274:149–154, 1995

Volpe JJ: Effect of cocaine use on the fetus. N Engl J Med 327:399–407, 1992

Warner LA, Kessler RC, Hughes M, et al: Prevalence and correlates of drug use and dependence in the United States. Arch Gen Psychiatry 52:219–228, 1995

11

General Hospital
and Primary Care Settings

General clinical settings, which range from school nurse offices to outpatient clinics to inpatient hospital units, are equally important in the detection, recognition, and treatment of substance use disorders (SUDs). It has been estimated that nearly half of all primary care patients have some type of problem related to substances (Miller and Gold 1998) and that 25%–50% of general hospital admissions are related to complications of substance use (Moore et al. 1989). This chapter is intended most for clinicians with primary responsibility in general clinical settings and health care providers consulting to those settings.

The General Hospital

A high index of suspicion may help the health care provider to detect a hidden SUD. There may be further advantages in confronting the addictive process during a medical crisis, when denial may be lessened or can be easily confronted by irrefutable medical evidence. Alcoholism may be diagnosed by associated medical problems such as liver disease, pancreatitis, anemia, certain types of pneumonia, delirium, dementia, gastric ulcers, esophageal varices, tuberculosis, or symptoms that mimic psychiatric syndromes.

The Outpatient Medical Setting

Outpatient settings such as primary care providers and outpatient specialty clinics, and nonmedical settings such as school nurse offices or others, have less capacity than inpatient settings to gather enough facts about the patient (e.g., those typically obtained through laboratory studies) to conduct an adequate assessment and address concerns about ensuring compliance and abstinence during a detoxification. But outpatient settings have the highest potential for finding cases and appropriately treating them. Many forms of detoxification, including that of opioids, can be performed by knowledgeable practitioners in such settings. Although assessment and treatment of SUDs by primary care physicians is growing, such patients are often in the care of psychiatrists as well. Outcomes in primary care buprenorphine practices may be similar to those found in specialized clinics (Stein et al. 2005). In many cases, the outpatient physician does not require the substance use expert's consultation at all.

Psychiatric Consultation to General Floors and the Emergency Department

Requests for consultations from general hospital floors may represent a straightforward need for substance abuse evaluation or more cryptic requests for evaluation of organicity, mood disorders, or acting-out behavior. Consultations may be requested for help in treating overdose or withdrawal, making an initial diagnosis, engaging patients in the therapeutic process, evaluating pain medications, advising on the treatment of trauma and burn patients or of pregnant substance abusers, and performing assessments for transplant. Often, SUD patients are perceived by house staff as being manipulative, demanding, and unappreciative, and in reality they can present as such. It is important not to disavow the staff's real feelings but instead provide a framework of understanding about the addictive process that can make these feelings meaningful and tolerable. The clinician's self-awareness of feelings induced by patients not only is diagnostic at times but also may relieve the guilt of having retaliatory fantasies. Few people go into medicine to dislike their patients. Having these feelings surface may be intolerable to some house staff. In affective illnesses, the presence of overwhelming affects may focus attention away from a concomitant addictive process. In cases of organicity, important historical information may simply be forgotten. Table 11–1 offers general guidelines for approaching this patient population.

Each consultation request should be reviewed in an attempt to ascertain most clearly what is being requested. Frequently, this requires a call to the referring physician. Questions of confidentiality may arise with patients regarding their substance abuse. Generally, confidentiality must be discussed and handled appropriately. Because honesty is one of the core treatment tools in an addictive disease process, conspiracies or secrets regarding substance abuse are not advisable.

Assessing the Chart

For a consultant, reviewing the medical chart in detail is essential, not only to pick up important information about admitting signs and symptoms, third-party statements, and mental status, but also to put together divergent clues of substance abuse in a fresh manner. Pertinent laboratory work, X rays, electroencephalograms (EEGs), computed tomography (CT) scans, and the like should be reviewed. Suggestions for additional laboratory work (e.g., magnesium levels in a patient with a history of delirium tremens) should be made.

Table 11–1. General considerations in approach to consultation

Maintain a high suspicion for drug abuse and obtain collected data.

Obtain serum and urine toxicology screens as soon as possible upon admission.

Know general principles of detoxification and its differential therapeutics.

Realize that detoxification must often be tailored to the individual patient.

Recall that when treating polysubstance dependence, sedative withdrawal occurs first.

Use challenge tests or estimate conservatively when considering initial detoxification dosages.

Recognize drug–drug interactions and effects of medications on mental status exam.

Always differentiate psychopathology, substance-induced disorders, and medical disorders.

The Interview

If the consult request includes a request for assessment of a substance abuse problem, this should be clearly stated to the patient early in the interview. The referring physician can be asked to join the interview if it seems appropriate. In writing up findings, it is best to briefly note the reason for the consultation, the patient's identifying information, and a concise history of present illness, past history, medical complications, medications, and mental status. The impressions and recommendations should be prominent and the focus of the consult. Often, this report is the only one read.

Treatment Planning

Specific recommendations for treatment range from outpatient substance abuse treatment to no further intervention or from inpatient substance abuse to psychiatric treatment. Active treatment must frequently be postponed until the acute medical problems are stabilized. For patients showing early abuse patterns, simple counseling, education, and appropriate reassurance may be all that is necessary. If the patient does not have marked medical or psychiatric complications, is motivated, does not have a serious abuse pattern, and has little prior treatment exposure, outpatient referral is preferable. Inpatient psychiatric treatment may be indicated when major psychiatric illnesses need to be treated (e.g., psychosis, major depression) or when the patient presents with suicidal or homicidal ideation. Many units for mentally ill, chemically abusing individuals have been created to treat the substance abuse patient with major psychiatric problems. Transfer to an inpatient rehabilitation unit, when indicated, should be a direct transfer from the hospital to the treatment facility. All detoxification regimens should be clearly and explicitly spelled out. It may be necessary to work with the treatment staff to modify regimens in case of medical complications such as liver or renal disease.

Additional Treatment Issues

It is important to realize that abstinence in itself is not evidence of satisfactory treatment. A patient can be free of drug or alcohol use or craving while in the hospital, but may quickly return to active use on discharge. Family and individual education about substance abuse and assessment of the meaning of drugs or alcohol use in that person's life can begin in the hospital. Drug urine screens or alcohol Breathalyzer tests may need to be obtained for general hospital inpatients. Occasionally, patients will find methods to use substances even while in the hospital. These patients should be transferred to locked units where articles and people entering can be monitored for contraband. Early confrontation of continuing alcohol or drug use may clear up complicated diagnostic pictures.

Making the Referral to Specialty Care

It is often best that the patient make the initial call for specialty care. It is also important that all calls be made while in the hospital setting and that appointments be set before discharge. In cases where substance abuse treatment facilities are connected with the general hospital, in-house contact is advised, as is attendance at in-house meetings, such as Alcoholics Anonymous (AA), when feasible.

Issues in the Care of the Medical/Surgical Patient With a Substance Use Disorder

Attention to Detoxification

Some persons who have dependence on one substance or another become medical inpatients for problems that have little to do with their misuse, and the primary team fails to appropriately address the patient's impending withdrawal. Alcohol or sedative-hypnotic withdrawal implies at least physiological dependence, and careful attention to the risks of withdrawal is important. Unfortunately, in some centers, misguided practices remain in use, which either are insufficiently precise or fail to achieve detoxification. For example, some practitioners provide medical inpatients with decreasing amounts of alcoholic beverages, such as beer, which is available in some hospital formularies. Other clinicians caring for nonpsychiatric or non-substance-related issues will choose not to detoxify—asserting that they are supporting the patient's lifestyle choice—and allow a steady ingestion of beer, even obtaining periodic tests of blood alcohol levels! At a minimum, individuals dependent on substances who are inpatient medical or surgical patients should receive appropriate detoxification, education, and referral for substance abuse treatment.

Drug Interactions

Special attention to drug interactions is necessary in the general hospital setting. When first admitted, patients may have psychoactive drugs in their system that will adversely interact with prescribed medications. Alcohol interacts with other medications in various ways (Table 11–2). One interesting and important way in which it does so is by its bimodal effect on the cytochrome P450 (CYP) system. Initially, alcohol can inhibit the metabolism of other drugs, thus increasing serum levels of oral anticoagulants, diazepam, and phenytoin. But after chronic use, alcohol can induce CYP enzymes, leading to decreased levels of these medications. Thorazine, chloral hydrate, and cimetidine all inhibit alcohol dehydrogenase. Finally, alcohol increases the absorption of diazepam and the potency of all central nervous system depressants. One should always have easy access to and frequently consult a good handbook of drug–drug interactions (Table 11–3).

Table 11–2.   Medication interactions with alcohol

Disulfiram	Flushing, diaphoresis, vomiting, confusion
Oral anticoagulants	Increased effect with acute intoxication, decreased effect after chronic use
Antimicrobials	Minor disulfiram reaction
Sedatives, hypnotics, narcotics, antihistamines	Increased central nervous system depression
Diazepam	Increased absorption
Phenytoin	Increased anticonvulsant effect with acute intoxication; alcohol intoxication or withdrawal may lower seizure threshold after chronic alcohol abuse
Salicylates	Gastrointestinal bleeding
Chlorpromazine	Increased levels of alcohol, lowered seizure threshold
MAOIs	Adverse reactions to tyramine in some alcoholic beverages

Note.   MAOIs = monoamine oxidase inhibitors.

Table 11–3. Significant drug–drug/substance interactions

Substance	Substance	Interaction
Alcohol	SSRI/venlafaxine	Anecdotal reports of being "more" drunk, easier blackouts. Possible basis: increased 5-HT transport, decreased intoxication effects
Opioids	Fluoxetine, MAOIs	Death, fulminant reaction
Methadone	Any QTc-prolonging medication or condition (e.g., many antipsychotic medications or hypokalemia)	Extension of QTc toward torsades de pointes
Methadone	Benzodiazepines	
Methadone, buprenorphine	Any medication that affects CYP3A4 enzyme activity	

Note. CYP = cytochrome P450; 5-HT = 5-hydroxytryptamine (serotonin); MAOIs = monoamine oxidase inhibitors; SSRI = selective serotonin reuptake inhibitor.

Management of Pain

Iatrogenic contributions to addiction are a major concern in treating substance abuse patients in the general hospital setting. These contributions are most notable in intravenous drug addicts for whom pain medication is required. Many staff members are trained to be very cautious and suspicious when prescribing pain medication for these patients. Excessive caution can lead to undermedication. Patients may present with low frustration tolerance, anxiety, demanding behavior, and manipulation. It must be stressed, however, that these patients do experience pain. If offensive patients provoke too much rage and anger in the staff, treatment personnel may be unconsciously driven to punish such patients by undermedicating them. In certain individuals, larger than usual doses of pain medications are indicated due to tolerance. Each patient should be evaluated carefully; history, pattern of abuse, personality, and physical pathology should be considered. When a substance abuse patient's concerns and requests are categorically dismissed, serious prejudicial attitudes among staff may be evident. In some cases, staff should remove themselves from the patient's care before a spiral develops that will end in the abandonment of the patient. Approximately one-quarter to one-third of patients receiving pain management with opioids are susceptible to opioid use disorder, especially dependence. It should be noted that the starting dose for methadone for pain has been reduced to avoid overdoses.

Chronic pain patients have a high profile for abusing drugs. Maintaining continuity of care and promoting realistic expectations are prominent treatment goals in this population. Clinicians need to devote time to using scales to score/quantify pain to validate pain complaints, to identify any associated psychiatric issues (or the denial thereof), to the patient's sense of being unique and the patient's fears of never being helped. It is necessary to avoid intramuscular medication and as-needed (prn) dose scheduling and to ensure adequate coverage (i.e., selection of medications that have adequate half-lives for dosage scheduling, appropriate administration, and the right medication for the type of pain) (Bouckoms and Hackett 1997). Furthermore, it is essential to ensure that adjuvant medications are used, ranging from tricyclic antidepressants to various mood stabilizers such as gabapentin, while maintaining awareness of the organ damage that may have been independently created by substances.

Cannabis/Cannabinoids for General Medical Conditions

Notwithstanding its dynamic legal status, cannabinoids, or medications that act at the cannabinoid receptor, have emerged, as well as cannabis itself, as substances used in the treatment of various chronic conditions, particularly those that include pain or nausea. The risks of this practice may outweigh the potential benefits. Frequently, those who actually use cannabis have a higher rate of preexisting psychiatric disorder—and this cannot be beneficial in the treatment of long-term neurological disorders such as multiple sclerosis (Arnett 2008).

Burn Patients

Use of alcohol and other substances is a risk factor for burns, and preburn use of these substances implies a worse prognosis for the burn patient: alcohol is an independent predictor of death in such patients (McGill et al. 1995). Burn patients who use alcohol or other substances require heightened attention from psychiatric and substance use standpoints, both in coping with present loss and in treatment planning for the future.

Organ Transplants

Increasing numbers of organ transplants will be performed in the coming years. Mental health personnel will be asked to assess patients' psychological readiness to receive such transplants. In developing criteria for eligibility for heart or liver transplants, alcoholism must be considered a complicating factor. Active alcoholism has been a contraindication for liver transplantation, although controversy surrounds this issue. The issue of evaluating recovering alcoholics is complicated. It has been estimated that up to one-half of all cases of hepatic failure in the United States are due to alcohol. Care must be taken not to discriminate against a stable recovering alcoholic who may well be a good candidate for transplant. The fear of relapse, which would undermine the benefits of this treatment, is a consideration; however, careful evaluation and application of certain criteria may diminish this risk. Such criteria might include at least 6 months of sobriety from alcohol, no other active substance abuse, and good family support. The recovering alcoholic may be able to be evaluated in line with other candidates. In fact, there is evidence that organ and patient survival rates among selected recovering alcoholics who receive transplants are as good as those for patients who receive livers for non-alcohol-related diseases (Berlakovich et al. 1994).

Sexually Transmitted Diseases

Various substances produce disinhibition or are associated with cultures that allow for high degrees of risky sexual contact, and this circumstance makes substance use reduction a high priority in reducing the transmission of human immunodeficiency virus (HIV) and other sexually transmitted diseases. In women with borderline personality disorder, the presence of a SUD significantly increases the risk of transmission of a major sexually transmitted disease (including gonorrhea, herpes, HIV, trichomonas, human papillomavirus, or syphilis) (Chen et al. 2007). Increased testing continues to be advocated, especially among those seeking substance use treatment. Those at greatest risk for HIV or for hepatitis C virus are injection drug users.

Key Points

- Pain should be sufficiently, although carefully, treated in all patients, including those with substance use disorders.
- Clinicians of all specialties should maintain the attitude that addiction is a disease that deserves intervention.
- Substances of abuse can affect medical conditions as well as the medications used to treat them.
- Misuse of substances can increase the risk of certain medical conditions.
- Withdrawal from alcohol or sedative-hypnotics can be fatal and requires appropriate attention.

References

Arnett PA: Cannabis bliss? Neurology 71:160–161, 2008

Berlakovich GA, Steininger R, Herbst F, et al: Efficacy of liver transplantation for alcoholic cirrhosis with respect to recidivism and compliance. Transplantation 58:560–565, 1994

Bouckoms A, Hackett TP: Pain patients, in Massachusetts General Hospital Handbook of General Hospital Psychiatry, 4th Edition. Edited by Cassem NH, Stern TA, Rosenbaum JF, et al. St Louis, MO, Mosby-Yearbook Publishing, 1997, pp 367–415

Chen EY, Brown MZ; Lo TT, et al: Sexually transmitted disease rates and high-risk sexual behaviors in borderline personality disorder versus borderline personality disorder with substance use disorder. J Nerv Ment Dis 195:125–129, 2007

McGill V, Kowal-Vern A, Fisher SG: The impact of substance use on mortality and morbidity from thermal injury. J Trauma 38:931–934, 1995

Miller NS, Gold MS: Management of withdrawal syndromes and relapse prevention in drug and alcohol dependence. Am Fam Physician 58:139–146, 1998

Moore RD, Bone LR, Geller G, et al: Prevalence, detection, and treatment of alcoholism in hospitalized patients. JAMA 261:403–407, 1989

Stein MD, Cioe P, Friedmann PD: Buprenorphine retention in primary care. J Gen Intern Med 20:1038–1041, 2005

12

Treatment Modalities

Psychosocial Modalities

Treatment is not simply "counseling." Cognitive-behavioral therapy, interpersonal therapy, dialectical behavior therapy, motivational interviewing, and psychodynamically oriented psychotherapy are important treatment modalities for substance use disorders (SUDs), although their benefit is often delayed. There are data that show that psychotherapy combined with certain psychopharmacological treatments is more efficacious than either alone (Carroll et al. 2004). On the other hand, there are some situations in which medication is absolutely needed.

Individual Therapy

Individual therapy can be conducted alone or with other modalities, including pharmacotherapy, 12-Step programs, and family and group treatments. Abstinence is an important measure of efficacy and should be considered a goal and a means to treatment success. Treatments range from psychodynamically informed, supportive, and expressive treatment to cognitive, behaviorally oriented treatment. Individual treatments are especially indicated when patients face bereavement, loss, or social disruption and have targeted problems (e.g., anxiety disorders, panic disorder). Brief interventions are sometimes effective and worth a try, especially in primary care settings; however, many patients require long-term care and follow-up.

Initiating Individual Treatment: The Therapeutic Contract

At the outset, the therapist should concentrate on whether the patient can accept that he or she has a problem and needs treatment in order to achieve and maintain sobriety. The contract between the patient and the therapist should address treatment frequency and modality, limit setting regarding continuation of treatment despite continued use, inclusion of significant others in the social network, a clear goal of abstinence, psychopharmacological treatment if indicated, and arrangements regarding costs and scheduling.

Individual Psychotherapies

Cognitive-behavioral therapy.   Cognitive-behavioral therapy has been modified for SUDs. The assumption is that abuse of and dependence on substances are learned behaviors and can be changed. Cognitive-behavioral therapy is a treatment in which the patient works to identify and modify maladaptive thought patterns, which lead to feelings that lead to use. Cognitive-behavioral therapy is very helpful for relapse prevention, as well as for patients who are dependent or sociopathic or who show symptoms of a primary psychiatric disorder. It has been helpful for prevention of relapse to cocaine. For depressed women who are also alcoholic, successful outcomes have been shown with a combination of sertraline and cognitive-behavioral therapy (Linehan et al. 1999). Cognitive-behavioral therapy also is used in combination with aversive therapies such as disulfiram (Carroll et al. 2004).

Dialectical behavior therapy.   Dialectical behavior therapy is a comprehensive, behaviorally oriented treatment designed for highly dysfunctional patients meeting criteria for borderline personality disorder. Many of these criteria describe characteristics of drug abuse patients and some of the problems encountered in treatment of drug abuse patients, especially when various treatments are combined. The basic challenge of the dialectical behavior therapist is the balancing of validation and acceptance treatment strategies with problem-solving procedures, including contingency management, exposure-based procedures, cognitive modification, and skills training. Dialectical behavior therapy has been shown to be more effective than treatment-as-usual in treating drug abuse in women with borderline personality disorder (Linehan et al. 1999).

Motivational interviewing and motivational enhancement therapy. Motivational enhancement therapy assumes that a patient is responsible for and capable of changing his or her behavior, and the motivational enhancement therapist focuses on helping a patient mobilize his or her own inner resources. The basic motivational principles utilized in motivational enhancement therapy are expression of empathy, the development of discrepancy, avoiding argumentation, rolling with resistance, and supporting self-efficacy. Motivation for change is developed by eliciting self-motivational statements, listening with empathy, questioning, presenting personal feedback, affirming the patient, handling resistance, and reframing. Motivational enhancement therapy is a specific application of motivational interviewing that was developed for use in the treatment of alcohol abuse. In this brief, two- to four-session treatment approach, counselors first guide patients through an examination of the pros and cons of their drug use (a "decisional balance") and of the difference between where they are and where they want to be, in an attempt to lead them to state their desire to change—the first step in recovery. Counselors then strengthen patients' commitment to change by helping them to identify their goals for recovery and to determine ways to reach these goals. Motivational interviewing can be used as a stand-alone counseling approach, but more often it is used as a first step in the recovery process, followed by other interventions. It can also be incorporated into subsequent treatment sessions to bolster patients' motivation as needed (Substance Abuse and Mental Health Services Administration 1999). At the right "stage" of recovery, the contribution of primary care motivational intervention is potentially great, and such intervention should be pursued by generalists (Schwartz et al. 2006; Hernandez-Avila et al. 1998).

Apart from formal motivational interviewing and motivational enhancement therapy, it should be noted that the *transtheoretical model* has become the cornerstone of treatment approaches to many medical problems in addition to addictions. "Readiness to change" is equivalent to motivation. Its presence predicts success in many populations (Joe et al. 1998). It is important to assess the stage in which the person sits at any time. The stages include precontemplation, contemplation, preparation, action, and maintenance (DiClemente et al. 2004).

Psychodynamically oriented therapy. Psychodynamically oriented individual treatment is for patients with problems in identity, separation and individuation, affect regulation, self-governance, and self-care. For those with addictive disorders and other neurotic problems, psychodynamically oriented therapy requires psychological mindedness; capacity for honesty, intimacy, and identification with the therapist; average-to-superior intelligence; economic stability; high motivation; and a willingness to discuss conflict. In patients with these characteristics, expressive psychotherapy may lead to deepening of a capacity to tolerate depression and anxiety without substance use. When patients are not abstinent, exploratory treatment may do more harm than good, with reactivation of painful conflicts leading to further drinking and regression (O'Connor et al. 1995). Formal psychoanalysis is contraindicated in early phases of addictive treatment, especially for patients who are actively drinking. Once abstinence has been achieved, however, some patients respond well to insight-oriented psychotherapy.

Couples Therapy

One type of couples therapy, behavioral couples therapy, has positive effects on substance abuse and improves relationship adjustments, including parenting (Winters et al. 2002). Recent evidence has shown decreased substance use as well as increased marital happiness as a result of behavioral couples therapy, and reduction in the level of domestic violence in couples where both partners are using (Fals-Stewart et al. 2006).

Group Therapy

Group therapy is frequently the principal treatment modality for addictive disorders. Groups provide opportunities for resocialization, practicing of social skills and object relatedness, and impulse control; they foster the patient's identity as a recovering person and support acceptance of abstinence. Groups support self-esteem and reality testing. Groups for addicted patients have the advantage of using the shared issue of dealing with addictions as a jumping-off point to discuss other problems that may be shared.

A variety of group formats have been found useful, including assertiveness training groups; couples groups; and groups for fostering self-control, enhancing ego strength and self-concept, and dealing with mood problems (e.g., anxiety, depression). Groups may be used to help in problem solving, to focus on specific behavioral problems, and to help the patient see that others have similar problems. They may be psychodynamically oriented, problem-solving, network, or confrontational; they may offer couples therapy or occupational counseling. Treatment programs frequently employ orientation-didactic groups, which may aid retention in treatment, promote cohesiveness, and support acceptance of longer-term rehabilitation. Although groups have primarily been used for persons with alcoholism, they may be especially effective for relapse prevention among individuals with cocaine dependence.

Addiction recovery groups emphasize the motto of "no drinking, no drugging, no matter what." The "no matter what" is the hard part, and the group focus is on increased self-care, self-esteem, and improved coping skills, other than the use of substances. Groups help to reduce stigma and provide solid role models and mutual help. Transference issues are different in groups than in individual therapy. Craving, slips, and the need to get back "on track" are discussed openly in group.

Network Therapy

In network therapy, a support group is developed that is tailored to the patient, involving family and friends who are not addicted themselves. Network therapy takes a cognitive-behavioral therapy approach regarding triggers and uses community reinforcement; support of the patient's social network is essential (Fiore et al. 2008). It can be a useful adjunct to individual therapy or Alcoholics Anonymous (AA) and involves provision of psychoeducation about addictions to the patient's circle of supports.

Family Evaluation and Therapy

A family evaluation is warranted for all SUD patients; information and aid from the family is crucial for both diagnosis and treatment. Family members frequently are greatly affected by the patient's problems. Often, the family system has been made to accommodate the patient's drinking and may to some degree reinforce it. Confrontation by family members in many cases represents the stimulus for the patient's initially seeking treatment and may be important in helping the patient remain in treatment.

Family treatment is frequently indicated, especially in families in which considerable support is available to the patient. The children of alcoholic patients may benefit from family evaluation and treatment. Family treatments based on the concept of the "alcoholic system" focus on correction of dysfunctional patterns of interactional behavior within the family; success is measured not only as achievement of abstinence by the patient but also as improvement of the level of functioning in the family. Modalities used by family therapists include conjoint family therapy, marital therapy groups, and conjoint hospitalization for marital couples. The efficacy of these interventions has been documented (American Psychiatric Association 1995).

Self-Help

Clinicians must be thoroughly familiar with the 12-Step self-help programs—AA, Al-Anon, Narcotics Anonymous (NA), Cocaine Anonymous, Gamblers Anonymous, and Overeaters Anonymous (including the personal experience of having attended meetings of both AA and Al-Anon)—so as to be in touch with their patients' experiences. A growing body of evidence has documented the efficacy of AA. Self-help may also be very important for cocaine abuse and dependence. Peer-led groups have been useful as well (Prochaska et al. 2004).

AA was formed in 1935 by Bill Wilson and Dr. Robert Smith in Akron, Ohio, in part due to lack of available medical treatment for alcoholism. It had roots in the Oxford movement (later the moral rearmament movement) and a Jungian emphasis on spirituality; it has grown into an international network that includes more than 2 million members in the United States and 185,000 groups worldwide. The major message of the organization is that people with alcohol problems, through recognition of alcoholism as an illness, can achieve sobriety together in a spiritual program that includes accepting powerlessness over alcohol and dependency through some intervention beyond the self. It is a voluntary, self-supporting fellowship that avoids any self-serving political or economic activity. Agnostics and atheists are welcome in 12-Step groups and can choose a "higher power" other than God—such as the AA group itself or a sponsor. Al-Anon is a program parallel to AA that includes self-help for the family. Other family-oriented programs include Alateen, for teenage users and teenage children of alcoholics, and groups for adult children of alcoholics.

How It Works

A 12-Step program involves a series of steps and traditions that rely heavily on self-honesty, sobriety, group process, humility, provision of successful role models, self-care, and destigmatization of alcoholism as an illness. Although a 12-Step program is frequently recommended in conjunction with a variety of other treatment approaches, for many patients the program may suffice as the sole treatment for an SUD. On average, members attend approximately 4 meetings per week, although in the early stages of involvement many attend 90 meetings in 90 days. Patients with multiple addictions may attend several different 12-Step programs. A variety of types of meetings include open ones that the interested public may attend, closed meetings, beginners' meetings, discussion groups, and homogeneous groups. Although groups vary in style, most generally have a warm, family feel and foster a sense of acceptance, mutual help, and understanding. The assumption is that alcoholics intuitively understand and can identify with universal problems faced by other alcoholics and can share feelings in a group. An emphasis on mutual help through helping others with the same problem has contributed widely to the success of this group, and a large part of the spirituality of the program is embedded in the generosity in time and energy of its members. A system of sponsorship of members by veteran AA attendees and the creation of a support network of exchanged telephone numbers are important aspects of AA membership. AA provides an opportunity for people to practice relatedness, gain structure, test values and judgment, exercise honesty, find acceptance, and regain hope.

The mechanism of effect of AA includes continuing exposure to the meetings. It is unknown if degree of participation is also related to effect (Moos and Moos 2004).

New Developments in Self-Help/12-Step Programs

Although AA began solely for individuals with alcoholism and originally was mostly composed of white middle-class men, in recent years many people get help earlier in their illness, and many more members are women. An expansion into a younger population, with more dual addiction and with additional psychiatric problems, has led to greater attention to these groups and their specific needs. Subgroups have developed for alcoholics who are gay or lesbian, physicians, adult children of alcoholics, atheists and agnostics, human immunodeficiency virus (HIV) positive, and those with dual diagnosis. Meetings can be found in major cities throughout the world and are essential for alcoholics who travel.

Referrals to 12-Step Programs

The therapist may take an active role in referring to 12-Step programs in addition to monitoring and interpreting resistance to regular attendance. The physician can have the patient call AA directly from the office or may call for the patient in order to select a meeting. A phone number (or Web site) for an AA intergroup is easily obtainable, and volunteers are glad to provide information about AA. Clinicians should address concerns or negative responses felt by patients on their first AA meetings. Initially, patients may have difficulties understanding AA or they may be socially avoidant. Patients with reactions to the spirituality of AA or those who feel criticized in AA because of their use of psychiatric medications or not accepted because of polysubstance abuse will need explanations and support. Patients should be encouraged to obtain an AA sponsor.

Contingency Management

Among the behavioral treatments centered on operant conditioning, contingency management has gained popularity as a treatment. Patients receive predetermined consequences (such as monetary-based incentives) contingent on achieving a therapeutic goal. Contingency management is useful in the rehabilitative care for dependence or abuse of many substances. For some populations of remitted cocaine-dependent individuals, it is equivalent in effect to cognitive-behavioral therapy. It is not necessarily helpful to combine cognitive-behavioral therapy with contingency management (Rawson et al. 2002). Nicotine dependence is an example of a condition that may be affected by contingency management (Higgins et al. 2004), given that it has been shown to be more effective than vouchers in reducing use among pregnant smokers. Contingency management has also been demonstrated to be effective in reducing methamphetamine use (Roll et al. 2006).

Counseling

Certified alcohol and drug counselors have increasingly played prominent roles in alcohol and drug treatment programs. They are involved in every phase of treatment, including evaluation, psychoeducation, individual and group counseling, and aftercare. For relapse prevention, counselors frequently provide support, advice, and valuable information regarding treatment and 12-Step programs.

Education

Most programs include education about alcohol and drugs effects, effects on the family, treatment alternatives, and relapse prevention. Education reduces fear, guilt, and shame; supports the medical model; and provides hope. Lectures, discussion groups, films, books, and homework assignments are an important part of the work of treatment and help keep patients productively engaged during treatment.

Case Management

Case managers provide the opportunity to ensure that the entire treatment plan is tailored to the individual patient. Functions of the case manager include fostering the interaction among the various roles, which include assessment, planning, linkage, monitoring, and advocacy. Issues such as transportation, child care, or housing needs are some of the services offered. When there are co-occurring disorders, case managers can be extremely helpful (Substance Abuse and Mental Health Services Administration 1998).

Spirituality and Recovery

For many patients, spiritual faith and belief systems can play a positive role in recovery and should be encouraged by clinicians. Clinicians should be continually sensitive to and competent in exploring this important aspect of patients' lives.

Pharmacological Modalities

In a multimodal treatment plan for an SUD there are several uses for pharmacological agents, including detoxification via short-term, tapered drug substitution (e.g., methadone, benzodiazepines), treatment of comorbid psychiatric and medical disorders, relapse prevention through aversive treatment (e.g., disulfiram in alcoholics), or attenuation of craving or euphoria (e.g., acamprosate, naltrexone). Generally, medications are used as adjuncts to psychosocial treatment and education. Physicians should have a clear understanding of differential diagnosis and natural history of SUDs, limitations of medications, drug–drug interactions, and side effects.

Naltrexone

Naltrexone's original indication was in the prevention of opioid relapse. As a pure opioid receptor antagonist with a high affinity for the mu receptor, naltrexone displaces heroin, morphine, and methadone. Naltrexone causes withdrawal symptoms in those intoxicated by opioids, which is the reason protocols have been used to slowly begin treating with this medication in conjunction with outpatient clonidine for withdrawal (see Chapter 13, "Treatment Approaches"). Naltrexone's main indication is for daily relapse prevention, usually at 50 mg/day.

Notwithstanding the introduction of several new medications for alcohol relapse prevention, the superior efficacy of naltrexone for alcohol relapse prevention is well documented (Collins et al. 2005). It usually prevents relapse when it is given at 50 mg/day for 3 months. Opioid receptor functioning is thought to be related to the etiology of alcohol dependence. Opioid mu receptor antagonists decrease overall alcohol use, probably by blocking release of dopamine in the nucleus accumbens.

In the past decade, several studies have indicated that naltrexone is less efficacious than had previously been assumed (Krystal et al. 2001), but most research has supported the efficacy of naltrexone in alcohol dependence relapse prevention (Heinälä et al. 2001). Study results have varied in terms of the associated psychosocial treatment. Naltrexone's superiority compared with acamprosate was demonstrated in Project COMBINE (Anton et al. 2006). Naltrexone is metabolized by the hepatic system (and acamprosate by the kidneys). At this point, which patients are better off with which medication is not well established. Genetic markers for response to naltrexone have been established, and commercial availability of measuring them for prognosis of response to naltrexone are in the offing.

Experimental and new formulations include rapid and ultrarapid detoxification as well as injectable naltrexone, which is not U.S. Food and Drug Administration (FDA) approved for opioid treatment, but which can be highly effective for opioid addiction when regularly injected. Depot administration has benefits of leading to a long period of abstinence and can lead to fewer visits for monitoring progress. One problem is the situation of emergent pain control if needed, because opioid receptors are blocked by a reservoir of naltrexone in the body. In that case, intensive monitoring (e.g., in an emergency department or intensive care unit) would be needed in order to override the blockade. Otherwise, this medication has a good safety profile. Side effects also include nausea, which usually lasts just a few days and then subsides, and can be treated with antinausea medications (Comer et al. 2006).

Methadone

A synthetic opioid, methadone has a dose-dependent effect on concurrent use of opioids and cocaine, and high dosages (65 mg/day) may be needed to be most effective. A stable dose need not be altered except in the case of changes in pharmacokinetics due to emesis; use of phenytoin, rifampin, barbiturates, carbamazepine, or tricyclic antidepressants; heavy labor; or alcohol intoxication. Owing to the frequency of overdoses, the FDA-approved starting dose of methadone to be given for pain now is 20–30 mg, but the dose is limited by regulation to be no more than 30 mg (Substance Abuse and Mental Health Services Administration 2005). Any concurrent use of benzodiazepines and methadone should be closely monitored, especially if the individual has impaired liver function. Physicians need training in pain management and the risks and benefits of management with opioids. High-dose methadone sometimes causes testosterone deficiency and sexual dysfunction.

Methadone poses risks to cardiac conduction in the form of extension of the QTc time interval on electrocardiogram (ECG), potentially leading to torsades de pointes, which may be fatal. In addition to usual patient assessment and monitoring, collaboration with the patient's primary and cardiac caregivers is important.

L-alpha-acetylmethadol (LAAM) is a long-acting opioid agonist but has been withdrawn due to its adverse-effect profile, especially its cardiac effects. It should be noted that there are several governmental regulations that affect the provision of methadone in methadone clinics, many of which are explained in Treatment Improvement Protocol (TIP) Series TIP 43 (Substance Abuse and Mental Health Services Administration 2005).

Buprenorphine

Buprenorphine (the sublingual form of the parenteral analgesic Buprenex) is a synthetic mixed-opioid agonist–antagonist that is effective in the treatment of opioid dependence (Substance Abuse and Mental Health Services Administration 1999). Many patients with opioid addiction who have been helped by this medication in outpatient settings after failing other treatments consider it a "miracle" drug. Buprenorphine in tablet form is marketed as Subutex. Suboxone, a buprenorphine/naloxone 4:1 combination sublingual tablet, is approved for use in opioid detoxification and maintenance. The naloxone in the tablet discourages illegal/injection street use because it precipitates withdrawal when administered intravenously (it is not bioavailable after oral ingestion). There have been anecdotal reports of antidepressant effects of Suboxone.

Some important points about buprenorphine include that it is safer in overdose, owing to its ceiling effect (Umbricht et al. 2004). A person using it does not achieve typical opioid-induced euphoria. It blocks other opioids. Buprenorphine is actually the only opioid to act on the ORL-1/orphanin nociceptive receptor; it also is not sedating. It is a partial agonist at the mu opioid receptor and an antagonist at the kappa receptor. With its high affinity and low intrinsic activity at the mu receptor, it will displace morphine, methadone, and other full opioid agonists. No one should receive naltrexone concurrently with buprenorphine. Buprenorphine is metabolized by cytochrome P450 (CYP) 3A4, so caution should be exercised in dosing and in conjunction with other substrates that affect CYP3A4 availability.

One study demonstrated that both alone and in combination with naloxone, buprenorphine was reinforcing among prior opioid addicts, meaning that it serves as a substance of abuse for such patients and, therefore, there is indeed a need to be concerned about diversion (Comer and Collins 2002). Reform of the legislation on buprenorphine has increased the number of patients for whom a practitioner may prescribe from 30 to 100. Unfortunately, many institutional and workplace policies bar dependent patients from returning to work while taking this medication. There is potential for drug–drug interactions when combined with central nervous system depressants, such as benzodiazepines. Adverse effects are usually mild and include those symptoms seen with other opioids. For use as a maintenance medication, dosing should initially be at 4 mg with a repeat at 1–2 hours. The dose should be adapted to reduce craving. The average daily dosage is 16 mg/day; few patients require more than 24 mg/day. Naloxone is not recommended in pregnancy; its safety is unknown in lactation, in hepatic impairment or geriatric cases, and in patients with pain, given that it blocks receptors. In cases with substantial other medication therapy, such as in individuals with HIV, this medication should be used with great caution. In all of these situations, one must remember that Suboxone includes two medications (buprenorphine and naloxone), and the risks of naloxone must be considered. A transition from methadone maintenance to buprenorphine maintenance should be carefully planned and should include consideration of the appropriate dose of buprenorphine.

Disulfiram

Disulfiram (Antabuse) is a medication adjunct in the treatment of recovering alcoholics. It is used as aversive treatment to enhance motivation for continued abstinence by making the high unavailable, thus discouraging impulsive alcohol use. Disulfiram is a potent reversible aldehyde dehydrogenase inhibitor. Aldehyde dehydrogenase is an enzyme that metabolizes acetaldehyde, the first metabolite of alcohol. Inhibition of this step produces a buildup of acetaldehyde, resulting in toxicity, which consists of nausea, vomiting, cramps, flushing, and vasomotor collapse. Disulfiram has relatively mild side effects, including sedation, halitosis, skin rash, and temporary impotence. More serious side effects, which include peripheral neuropathy, seizures, optic neuritis, or psychosis, occur rarely. Disulfiram also appears to have a catecholamine effect, which may contribute to the alcohol reaction and make its use contraindicated with monoamine oxidase inhibitor (MAOI) use. It may also inhibit the metabolism of other medications, including anticoagulants, phenytoin, and isoniazid, leading to higher-than-expected serum levels of these medications. The drug also has adverse interactions with cough syrups and other consumer products containing alcohol, such as mouthwash. Disulfiram should be avoided in patients who are pregnant and patients with hepatic disease, peripheral neuropathy, renal failure, or cardiac disease. Disulfiram should not be used for more than 1 year due to increased risk of peripheral neuropathy and liver problems. Other contraindications include medical conditions that would be greatly exacerbated by a disulfiram–alcohol reaction, including liver disease, esophageal varices, heart disease, heart failure, hypertension, emphysema, and peptic ulcer disease. It should be avoided in anyone likely to become pregnant. Psychiatric contraindications include psychosis and severe depression. Disulfiram can exacerbate psychosis; depressed suicidal patients may purposely precipitate a disulfiram reaction.

Initial dosages of disulfiram are 250–500 mg/day; it can be administered in an oral suspension. Subcutaneous implantation is not clinically available. Dosages can be adjusted downward to 125 mg/day if sedation or other side effects are excessive, or in those with relative contraindications. Patients should be informed about the rationale of disulfiram use, the disulfiram–alcohol reaction, and common side effects.

Treatment facilities vary in their use and attitudes toward disulfiram. Some AA-oriented programs may discourage the use of any medication and see disulfiram as an unnecessary psychopharmacological crutch. Many programs use disulfiram as an adjunctive tool in promoting abstinence. Although there has not been convincing evidence that disulfiram use affects long-term outcomes globally, disulfiram has been shown to be useful in certain situations, such as when it can be administered by a significant other. Socially stable adult alcoholics and affluent married patients with less sociopathy who tend to be compulsive do better on disulfiram. Compliance with disulfiram can be monitored by a spouse or employer.

Acamprosate

Acamprosate is a new medication with great promise in alcohol relapse prevention (Johnson et al. 2008). It crosses the blood–brain barrier, is chemically similar to amino acid neurotransmitters, and acts at the N-methyl-D-aspartate (NMDA) receptor to reduce withdrawal's glutaminergic hyperactivity. It is dose dependent and has no abuse potential. Giving acamprosate to those dependent on alcohol will not lead to an acute withdrawal syndrome. Acamprosate is not metabolized, but rather is renally excreted and should be given with caution to those with renal disease. A starting dosage is 2–3 g/day divided into three doses, and common side effects include diarrhea or headache. Acamprosate is metabolized by the kidneys. It may be combined with naltrexone for an even greater effect in reducing relapse (Kiefer et al. 2003). However, as a major focus of the COMBINE study (Anton et al. 2006), acamprosate did not add to the effectiveness of naltrexone.

Lithium

Lithium is an integral component in the treatment of SUDs with underlying primary bipolar or cyclothymic disorders. Lithium may mute or abort extreme mood swings or may indirectly affect substance intake. Mania or hypomania is associated with increased alcohol or cocaine use. Lithium-responsive depression may also be associated with cocaine or alcohol abuse. Lithium has also been associated with decreased subjective experience of intoxication, antagonization of deficits in cognitive and motor function during intoxication, and reduced alcohol consumption. Caution should be exercised in prescribing lithium to those who are actively abusing substances or those who demonstrate poor compliance with treatment. These patients need to be hospitalized to ensure abstinence and titration of a proper dose. There are no known uses of lithium in uncomplicated alcohol abuse or dependence. For adolescents with bipolar disorder and secondary substance dependence, lithium is efficacious for both disorders (Moak et al. 2003). Although lithium is dangerous in overdose, more than any other psychiatric medication it has proven results in reducing suicide in bipolar disorder.

Valproic Acid

Valproic acid is used in the treatment of bipolar disorder. Moderate doses of valproate (with an average blood level of approximately 70 mg/L) in alcoholics without significant hepatic disease do not cause significant adverse effects on white blood count, platelet count, or liver transaminase level (Carroll et al. 2004). There has been increasing interest in use of valproate in detoxification from alcohol. Patients with bipolar disorder and addictions tend to prefer other mood stabilizers to lithium, perhaps because of side-effect profiles such as tremor. Valproate given to patients with bipolar disorder who are dependent on alcohol reduces alcohol consumption (Salloum et al. 2005).

Antidepressants

Antidepressants do not directly alter SUDs but are important adjuncts in the treatment of patients with primary mood disorders. Determining the antidepressant of choice follows considerations of the depressive subtype and side-effect profile of the medications and recognition that judgment, impulse control, and cognition may be impaired with alcoholics in early recovery. Extreme caution should be used in placing alcoholics on MAOIs for depression, especially because wine contains tyramine. Also, intoxication may further impair judgment and increase the risk of using tyramine-containing products. There is evidence that fluoxetine is not helpful for primary cocaine dependence. Venlafaxine, a broad-spectrum antidepressant, may be a safe, well-tolerated, rapidly acting, and effective treatment for patients with a dual diagnosis of depression and cocaine dependence. Venlafaxine's potential to cause diastolic hypertension at higher doses indicates monitoring of blood pressure. Use of duloxetine (Cymbalta) for patients with pain and substance use could be useful.

Antidepressants, particularly bupropion, have been employed for smoking cessation. There is good evidence that bupropion is an effective aid for both adults and adolescents. Its mechanism of action is unknown.

Dopamimetics

Bromocriptine, a dopamine agonist, has been studied in the treatment of cocaine addiction. It had been hypothesized that because cocaine's effects are dopamine related, and because dopamine depletion is associated with cocaine craving, a dopamimetic substance such as bromocriptine may have some value in the acute onset of abstinence (first 3–4 days) by diminishing cocaine craving. But studies have failed to justify application of bromocriptine, and we do not recommend its use in cocaine SUDs. Similarly, amantadine has not been found to aid in cocaine dependence.

Clonidine

Clonidine's use in opioid detoxification is discussed in Chapter 13 ("Treatment Approaches"). Clonidine has also been reported to be helpful in alcohol withdrawal. There have been case reports of the successful use of clonidine for patients with hallucinogen persisting perception disorder (Linehan et al.

1999). Clonidine is capable of improving rates of cessation from nicotine, probably by dampening the withdrawal syndrome severity.

Carbamazepine

Carbamazepine, an anticonvulsant, has demonstrated efficacy in treating mild to moderate alcohol withdrawal. Although previously felt to be helpful for symptoms in abstinence from cocaine, more recent studies have failed to show carbamazepine to be an effective agent against cocaine (Substance Abuse and Mental Health Services Administration 1999).

Gabapentin

Gabapentin is not FDA approved for cocaine treatment. It has been used experimentally because it is reported to have positive effects on the reduction of cocaine use and the lengthening of cocaine-free periods (Raby and Coomaraswamy 2004)

Topiramate

Topiramate may be useful in decreasing drinking. It has been shown to decrease the primary aberration of excessive drinking by reducing the reinforcing effects of alcohol. Its mechanism may be the facilitation of γ-aminobutyric acid (GABA) through a nonbenzodiazepine site and the antagonism of glutamate activity at other receptors as well. A 17-site double-blind, randomized trial of topiramate showed that it reduced drinking and produced abstinence (as well as improving other indicators of health, such as body mass index, hepatic enzymes, plasma cholesterol, and blood pressure) (Johnson et al. 2008). At the same time, there is also an awareness that topiramate might be abused, especially because it promotes weight loss. Topiramate has substantial side effects, including mental confusion, and it is not yet FDA approved for alcoholism.

Adrenergic Blockers

Use of propranolol, a beta-blocker, to reduce adrenergic signs of alcohol withdrawal is controversial and not routinely advocated. Beta-blockers are contraindicated in cocaine intoxication and withdrawal.

Antipsychotics

Antipsychotics must always be used with care, and this is no less the case for individuals who have had exposure to substances of abuse. Antipsychotics have no place in the treatment of primary alcoholism. They lower seizure threshold and carry a long-term risk of tardive dyskinesia. However, they can be very helpful in treating psychosis across a wide spectrum of toxic drug reactions. Antipsychotics can be used adjunctively with benzodiazepines in the treatment of delirium, including delirium tremens. Among the second-generation antipsychotics, olanzapine appears to be as effective as haloperidol in the treatment of cannabis-induced psychotic disorder, and is associated with a lower rate of extrapyramidal symptoms (Berk et al. 1999). On the other hand, selection of a second-generation antipsychotic requires consideration of the risk of weight gain, alteration in lipid profile, diabetes, and disordered movements, and these should be monitored for all patients. Quetiapine has become popular for its soporific effects and may seem attractive for that purpose in patients who should not receive benzodiazepines, but its use as a soporific should be approached with caution. Antipsychotics are the mainstay of treatment for schizophrenia and, frequently, bipolar disorder. They are rarely used in the treatment of severe anxiety conditions.

Varenicline

Varenicline is a new agent used in nicotine cessation. It is an α_4, β_2 nicotine receptor partial agonist that utilizes a different mechanism than nicotine replacement therapy or bupropion. It has a slightly larger effect size than does nicotine replacement therapy or bupropion, with an odds ratio of 2.5–3.0 versus 2.0 for nicotine replacement therapy plus bupropion. Its cost remains an issue. It should be used with care and may cause nausea. One comparison study found cessation rates of 44%, 29.5%, and 17.7% with varenicline, bupropion, and placebo, respectively (Gonzales et al. 2006). The FDA has warned about neuropsychiatric symptoms, increased suicidal thinking, and exacerbations of preexisting psychiatric illness associated with its use, but the effects of the medicine itself are unclear in this regard and its effectiveness in helping patients to quit smoking often may outweigh the risks.

Benzodiazepines

Benzodiazepines are the treatment of choice for alcohol or benzodiazepine detoxification. They work through the GABA receptor and are very effective in suppressing anxiety symptoms. They also produce tolerance, with psychological and physical dependence. Benzodiazepines are generally contraindicated in any SUD except when used for detoxification, for manic patients acutely, or very selectively in compliant abstinent patients with anxiety disorders when other treatments have failed.

A common dilemma is faced when the SUD patient has an underlying anxiety disorder, often presenting with high-dose benzodiazepine abuse. These patients may have a relapse of symptoms on detoxification from central nervous system depressants. It is often difficult to distinguish symptoms of underlying disorders from anxiety symptoms associated with chronic subacute withdrawal, reactive fear, and anxiety about withdrawal. After detoxification, these patients may be extremely anxious and dysphoric. Temptations to relieve this suffering may lead clinicians to reinstate addictive substances, which can lead to a poor outcome. Alprazolam, in particular, can cause a rebound increase in anxiety that may lead to relapse of alcohol or substance use or escalation of abuse. Effective utilization of other, perhaps more specific, treatment modalities include selective serotonin reuptake inhibitors (SSRIs), desipramine, or MAOIs for panic, and an antipsychotic for psychotic disorders, or SSRIs, buspirone, gabapentin, and adrenergic blockers for generalized anxiety. Setting firm limits on the use of psychoactive substances is necessary. Nonetheless, sometimes benzodiazepines can be a treatment of last resort in compliant patients with anxiety who maintain sobriety.

Buspirone

Buspirone (BuSpar) is an anxiolytic with no central nervous system depressant activity. Clinical studies have so far demonstrated little abuse potential or withdrawal syndrome. Buspirone apparently does not potentiate the effects of alcohol. This medication is a useful adjunct in the treatment of generalized anxiety or transient anxiety in some patients with SUDs. Buspirone has the disadvantage of slow onset of efficacy (up to 3 weeks); it is, thus, of little use in transient anxiety disorders.

Ondansetron

The selective serotonin 3 ($5\text{-}HT_3$) receptor antagonist ondansetron has shown promise in reducing alcohol intake in general, specifically among Type I alcoholic individuals, and in diminishing the subjective positive effects of alcohol. Its widespread use awaits further study.

Cannabinoids

Dronabinol is a synthetic form of delta-9-tetrahydrocannabinol. Case studies have highlighted its potential utility in cannabis-dependent patients (Levin and Kleber 2008).

Vaccines

Many investigators have studied the potential for vaccines as a part of the treatment of cocaine dependence. The studies have not led to positive results on the whole.

Key Points

- A wide array of treatment modalities have been used in the care of substance use disorders.
- Many studies have documented the superiority of treatments that combine psychosocial and pharmacological approaches over those that use exclusively one or the other modality.
- Clinicians should be wary of novel, unassessed treatment modalities.

References

American Psychiatric Association: Practice guideline for the treatment of patients with substance use disorders: alcohol, cocaine, opioids. Am J Psychiatry 152 (11 suppl): 1–59, 1995

Anton RF, O'Malley SS, Ciraulo DA, et al: Combined pharmacotherapies and behavioral interventions for alcohol dependence: the COMBINE study: a randomized controlled trial. JAMA 295:2003–2017, 2006

Berk M, Brook S, Trandafir AI: A comparison of olanzapine with haloperidol in cannabis-induced psychotic disorder: a double-blind randomized controlled trial. Int Clin Psychopharmacol 14:177–180, 1999

Carroll KM, Fenton LR, Ball SA, et al: Efficacy of disulfiram and cognitive behavioral therapy in cocaine-dependent outpatients: a randomized placebo-controlled trial. Arch Gen Psychiatry 61:264–272, 2004

Collins ED, Kleber HD, Whittington RA, et al: Anesthesia-assisted vs buprenorphine-or clonidine-assisted heroin detoxification and naltrexone induction: a randomized trial. JAMA 294:903–913, 2005

Comer S, Collins ED: Self-administration of intravenous buprenorphine and the buprenorphine/naloxone combination by recently detoxified heroin abusers. J Pharmacol Exp Ther 303:695–703, 2002

Comer SD, Sullivan MA, Yu E, et al: Injectable, sustained-release naltrexone for the treatment of opioid dependence: a randomized, placebo-controlled trial. Arch Gen Psychiatry 63:210–218, 2006

DiClemente CC, Schlundt D, Gemmell L: Readiness and stages of change in addiction treatment. Am J Addict 13:103–119, 2004

Fals-Stewart W, Birchler GR, Kelley ML: Learning sobriety together: a randomized clinical trial examining behavioral couples therapy with alcoholic female patients. J Consult Clin Psychol 74:579–591, 2006

Fiore MC, Jaén CR, Baker TB, et al: Treating Tobacco Use and Dependence: 2008 Update. Clinical Practice Guideline. Rockville, MD, U.S. Department of Health and Human Services. 2008

Gonzales D, Rennard SI, Nides M, et al: Varenicline, an alpha4beta2 nicotinic acetylcholine receptor partial agonist, vs sustained-release bupropion and placebo for smoking cessation: a randomized controlled trial. JAMA 296:47–55, 2006

Heinälä P, Alho H, Kiianmaa K, et al: Targeted use of naltrexone without prior detoxification in the treatment of alcohol dependence: a factorial double-blind, placebo-controlled trial. J Clin Psychopharmacol 21:287–292, 2001

Hernandez-Avila CA, Ortega-Soto HA, Jasso A, et al: Treatment of inhalant-induced psychotic disorder with carbamazepine versus haloperidol. Psychiatr Serv 49:812–815, 1998

Higgins ST, Heil SH, Solomon LJ, et al: A pilot study on voucher-based incentives to promote abstinence from cigarette smoking during pregnancy and postpartum. Nicotine Tob Res 6:1015–1020, 2004

Joe GW, Simpson DD, Broome KM: Effects of readiness for drug abuse treatment on client retention and assessment of process. Addiction 93:1177–1190, 1998

Johnson BA, Rosenthal N, Capece JA, et al: Improvement of physical health and quality of life of alcohol dependent individuals with topiramate treatment. Arch Intern Med 168:1188–1199, 2008

Kiefer F, Jahn H, Tarnaske T, et al: Comparing and combining naltrexone and acamprosate in relapse prevention of alcoholism: a double-blind placebo controlled study. Arch Gen Psychiatry 60:92–99, 2003

Krystal JH, Cramer JA, Krol WF, et al: Naltrexone in the treatment of alcohol dependence. N Engl J Med 345:1734–1739, 2001

Levin FR, Kleber HD: Use of dronabinol for cannabis dependence: two case reports and review. Am J Addictions 17:161–164, 2008

Linehan MM, Schmidt H 3rd, Dimeff LA, et al: Dialectical behavior therapy for patients with borderline personality disorder and drug dependence. Am J Addict 8:279–292, 1999

Moak DH, Anton RF, Latham PK, et al: Sertraline and CBT for depressed alcoholics: results of a placebo-controlled trial. J Clin Pharmacol 23:553–562, 2003

Moos RH, Moos BS: Long term influence on duration and frequency of participation in Alcoholics Anonymous on individuals with alcohol use disorders. J Consult Clin Psychol 72:81–90, 2004

O'Connor PG, Waugh ME, Carroll KM, et al: Primary care-based ambulatory opioid detoxification: the results of a clinical trial. J Gen Intern Med 10:255–260, 1995

Prochaska JJ, Delucci K, Hall SM, et al: A meta analysis of smoking cessation interventions with individuals in substance abuse treatment or recovery. J Consult Clin Psychol 72:1144–1156, 2004

Raby WN, Coomaraswamy S: Gabapentin reduces cocaine use among addicts from a community clinic sample. J Clin Psychiatry 65:84–86, 2004

Rawson RA, Huber A, McCann M, et al: A comparison of contingency management and cognitive-behavioral approaches during methadone maintenance treatment for cocaine dependence. Arch Gen Psychiatry 59:817–824, 2002

Roll JM, Petry NM, Stitzer ML, et al: Contingency management for the treatment of amphetamine use disorders. Am J Psychiatry 163:1993–1999, 2006

Salloum IM, Cornelius JR, Daley DC, et al: Efficacy of valproate maintenance in patients with bipolar disorder and alcoholism: a double-blind placebo-controlled study. Arch Gen Psychiatry 62:37–45, 2005

Schwartz RP, Highfield DA, Jaffe JH, et al: A randomized controlled trial of interim methadone maintenance. Arch Gen Psychiatry 63:102–109, 2006

Substance Abuse and Mental Health Services Administration, Center for Substance Abuse Treatment: Comprehensive Case Management for Substance Abuse Treatment. Treatment Improvement Protocol (TIP) Series 27. Rockville, MD, U.S. Department of Health and Human Services, 1998

Substance Abuse and Mental Health Services Administration, Center for Substance Abuse Treatment: Enhancing Motivation for Change in Substance Use Disorder Treatment. Treatment Improvement Protocol (TIP) Series 35. Rockville, MD, U.S. Department of Health and Human Services, 1999

Substance Abuse and Mental Health Services Administration, Center for Substance Abuse Treatment: Medication-Assisted Treatment for Opioid Addiction in Opioid Treatment Programs. Treatment Improvement Protocol (TIP) Series 43. Rockville, MD, U.S. Department of Health and Human Services, 2005

Umbricht A, Huestis MA, Cone EJ, et al: Effects of high dose intravenous buprenorphine in experienced opioid abusers. J Clin Psychopharmacol 24:479–487, 2004

Winters J, Fals-Stewart W, O'Farrell TJ, et al: Behavioral couples therapy for female substance-abusing patients: effects on substance use and relationship adjustment. J Consult Clin Psychol 70:344–355, 2002

13

Treatment Approaches

The clinician's response to a clinical presentation should be appropriate for the patient's particular presentation at the time. Interventions should be formulated in terms of attitudes, medications, psychotherapies, and setting/intensity. In this chapter, we review treatment for specific substance-related and substance-induced states, and we also consider medication and psychosocial treatments used for those states.

Abstinence

The importance of complete abstinence from all substances (except for maintenance replacement and substitution therapies) in the treatment of substance use disorders (SUDs) cannot be overestimated as a goal. The simplicity of "no drinking, no drugging, no matter what" must be communicated, along with an awareness of the patient's tendency to rationalize "one last use" in myriad ways. Partial abstinence, a lesser goal, does reduce morbidity and mortality and may be considered an improvement. Nevertheless, although many recovering patients want to continue using alcohol or other substances, it is impossible to identify those few for whom controlled use is safe. Total abstinence from all substances provides the best prognosis, and all treatment plans should include means to assess for relapse. Dual-diagnosis patients need to have medications—such as antipsychotics and antidepressants—continued even through relapse.

Recovery

The concept of abstinence is different from the concept of recovery or sobriety. Recovery implies a process in which the individual not only has ceased using drugs but also is actively developing a normal, balanced lifestyle, healthy self-esteem, and healthy intimacy in a sense of meaningful living. For addictive patients, recovery is a never-ending process; the term *cure* is avoided.

Relapse

What is relapse? Is it a return to the preabstinence level of substance use? Is it any use at all? Is it a loss of resolution toward changing abuse behavior? Is relapse only the active resumption of substance abuse, or can certain behaviors be labeled on a continuum in the process of relapse? Does the substitution of another form of addictive behavior (e.g., overeating, overworking, or gambling) constitute a relapse?

Relapse is a process of attitudinal change that usually results in reuse of alcohol or drugs after a period of abstinence. It is an important clinical phenomenon in the course of substance abuse treatment. In fact, addiction can be described as a disease characterized by recurrent relapses. More than 90% of patients in any one 12-month period after initiating abstinence will likely use substances; 45%–50% will return to pretreatment levels of morbidity (Armour et al. 1978). Thus, it is extremely important that those who have made commitments to recovery understand and anticipate relapse. They must develop coping strategies and contingency plans to thwart relapse, minimize the extent of damage, and promote renewed abstinence quickly.

Relapse Prevention

Relapse prevention is a vital part of the approach to anyone in remission. Cognitive-behavioral techniques are being used to successfully promote relapse prevention. The patient must understand his or her own unique set of high-risk relapse situations and avoid them or employ coping techniques to resist relapse when offered substances. Prior to relapse prevention training, what is stressed is a thorough understanding of one's self-motivational reasons for discontinuing addictive behavior, being able to work through alternative responses to situations, and choosing abstinence as part of the best mode of response. Marlatt and Gordon (1985) identified eight categories of high-risk drinking situations that could be applicable to other substance abuse: unpleasant emotions, physical discomfort, pleasant emotions, testing personal control, urges and temptations, conflict with others, social pressure to drink, and pleasant times with others. Which particular situation presents the highest risk can vary among individuals or drug classes. For example, young abusers may be most susceptible to relapse when experiencing positive feelings. Older, more chronic users may relapse more often due to depression or guilt. Abuse of opiates and cocaine may be more heavily tied to environmental cues. Adolescents may be more susceptible to peer pressure.

It is important to identify and watch for thoughts and feelings that typically occur during these high-risk situations. Homework assignments, complete with relapse prevention workbooks, teach patients the ins and outs of the relapse process, help them develop alternative coping skills, and reinforce the experience of a sense of self-mastery in these situations. Relapse prevention is especially valuable in outpatient settings where opportunities are present to practice skills in a natural environment. Behavioral techniques such as role-playing and assertiveness training are also valuable.

Guilt and Shame Reduction

The clinician expects the patient to see relapse neither as an "all or none" act nor as an unforeseeable or unavoidable event. Relapse, defined as a change in a resolution to change, is a fairly common experience that we all have at times. Relapse, then, is a fact of everyday life. Understanding this may prevent the patient's feeling that he or she has totally failed and that all is lost if a return to use occurs. Marlatt and Gordon (1985) coined the term "abstinence violation effect" to describe the view that once use occurs, it must inevitably lead to the pretreatment level of use. Guilt, shame, a sense of lack of control, trapped feelings, and lack of a prespecified plan may escalate substance use. The immediate benefit of substance use may overshadow the realization of the negative long-term consequences.

Practicing Social Skills

Identifying personal strengths, past coping behaviors, and environmental supports is important. Examples of alternative coping mechanisms when faced with temptation of substance use include calling a friend or sponsor, leaving the setting, or refusing the next drink. Relapse prevention may require, especially in the early stages of recovery, avoidance of high-risk situations and cues. Later on in the process, some avoidable high-risk situations can be mastered with alternative coping skills. Social skills training has also been used in prevention. In some situations, however, it may be advisable to avoid cues at all costs (e.g., having a "crack" addict not return to a setting where cocaine is being used).

Predictors of Successful Treatment Outcome

Seeking treatment following a diagnosis of a SUD is the first step—not everyone does it! Predictors of treatment seeking following assessment include late onset of disorder, using larger amounts than intended, unsuccessful attempts to decrease use, tolerance, the presence of withdrawal symptoms, and use of cocaine or heroin (Kessler et al 2001).

Treatment outcomes are better among individuals with high socioeconomic stability, low levels of antisocial personality, no comorbid psychiatric or medical problems, and a negative family history for alcoholism. History of contact with Alcoholics Anonymous (AA), stable work and marriage history, and fewer arrests are also correlated with better outcome. Most studies of treatment settings have not differentiated outcome by treatment setting, yet it is sicker patients who are more often hospitalized and stay longer. As a goal of therapy, remission is more difficult to achieve among patients who have polysubstance use, psychiatric symptoms, or significant emotional distress (Ritsher et al. 2002).

Differential Therapeutics

Although it is essential to engage patients in some therapy for as long as possible, the literature on differential therapeutics is limited. Despite developments in treatment outcome research, choosing the right treatment for a specific patient is still largely based on the conventional wisdom of clinical considerations. In selecting treatments or treatment combinations, the clinician should bear in mind that many patients have co-occurring psychiatric illness, that individuals frequently have multiple addictions, and that interventions should fit the unique needs of the patient (Compton et al. 2007). Other factors to be considered include presence of medical illness, severity of illness, individual patient characteristics (including cultural issues or concerns), availability of treatment resources, and awareness of the differential therapeutics of concomitant psychiatric disorders. Recent advances in biobehavioral approaches to psychiatric disorders (i.e., cognitive, behavioral, and psychodynamic individual approaches, and group and family treatment) need to be considered as well. Integration of 12-Step approaches such as AA or Narcotics Anonymous is also widely recommended.

One study in particular has demonstrated the importance of examining different modalities: the Combined Pharmacotherapies and Behavioral Interventions for Alcohol Dependence Study (COMBINE) is a multisite clinical trial initiated in 1997 to determine whether treatment for alcohol use disorders can be improved by combining pharmacotherapy and behavioral interventions (Anton et al. 2006).

Matching Treatments to Patients

In the past it was easy to apply the finding that longer inpatient stays were more likely to lead to full or partial abstinence from alcohol and reduced relapse rates on follow-up. Today, however, there are more treatment options and more pressure for efficiency. This trend is especially important for patients with SUDs and psychiatric disorders. In a series of classic studies, McLellan et al. (1997) found that matching a patient's problems with appropriate treatment services improves treatment effectiveness and leads to good overall effectiveness for alcohol treatment. Patients with severe psychiatric problems did poorly regardless of modality or treatment setting. Patients with legal problems did poorly in inpatient programs. Those with the least severe psychiatric problems did well in inpatient and outpatient settings. It was those patients whose psychiatric illness was in the middle range of severity *and* who also had employment or family problems that most needed inpatient care and that showed the greatest improvement when psychiatric services were also provided.

In terms of matching patients to detoxification settings, guidelines produced by the American Society of Addiction Medicine (ASAM) include five levels of care (Table 13–1); this system of levels has been widely applied, although its outcome validity is unknown (Mee-Lee et al. 2001). As always, placement should be according to the least restrictive alternative concept.

Treatment Settings

Inpatient

Inpatient treatment is indicated in the presence of major medical and psychiatric problems and their complications; severe withdrawal signs such as delirium tremens (DTs) or seizures; a history of failed trials of outpatient treatment; lack of an adequate social support network (family, friends, or AA members) for abstinence; or polysubstance addiction requiring inpatient management. In most other cases, a trial of outpatient treatment is indicated before hospitalization, unless there are complications. Patients prefer outpatient treatment, which is less disruptive and more cost-effective than inpatient treatment. Inpatient detoxification is followed by outpatient treatment or by inpatient rehabilitation.

The choice of inpatient rehabilitation in a freestanding substance recovery program, a freestanding inpatient psychiatric hospital, or a general hospital psychiatric unit depends on the severity of the patient's additional psychiatric and medical problems. Patients with the most severe psychiatric illness may need to be treated in a locked general hospital inpatient psychiatric unit before transfer to a mental illness/chemical abuse treatment unit.

Treatment outcome is related to treatment length, in that patients who complete day hospital substance abuse rehabilitation and then continue to participate in self-help groups are likely to have lower rates of alcohol and cocaine use during follow-up. Furthermore, the beneficial effect of self-help

Table 13-1. Detoxification setting levels defined by the American Society of Addiction Medicine

Level	Title	Description
Level I-D	Ambulatory detoxification without extended onsite monitoring	An organized outpatient service with preset assessment intervals
Level II-D	Ambulatory detoxification with extended onsite monitoring	Organized outpatient setting with service devoted to monitoring, such as day hospital
Level II.2-D	Clinically managed residential detoxification	24-hour support available, and peer and social support is emphasized
Level III.7-D	Medically monitored inpatient detoxification	24-hour medically supervised detoxification provided, as in freestanding detoxification center
Level IV-D	Medically managed intensive inpatient detoxification	24-hour acute care, as in inpatient psychiatric unit

Source.   Mee-Lee et al. 2001.

group participation does not appear to be strictly the result of motivation or some other patient characteristic.

Outpatient

The variety of outpatient settings is much larger than inpatient, ranging from the individual office practitioner or an addiction day or evening treatment program to the primary care provider. All may utilize techniques employed in inpatient treatment programs. Indications for outpatient alcohol detoxification include high motivation and good social support, no previous history of DTs or seizures, brief or nonsevere recent binges, no serious medical or psychiatric problems or polysubstance addiction, and prior successful outpatient detoxifications. Treatment for cocaine dependence in the community can also be efficacious; positive outcomes are correlated with level of treatment exposure and inversely related to magnitude of pretreatment use (Simpson et al. 2002).

Other Settings

Other settings in which substance use disorders are frequently treated include residential treatment programs, therapeutic communities, transitional residential programs/halfway houses, partial hospital/day treatment programs, and intensive outpatient programs.

Clinical Situations

Overdose

There are more than 5 million poisonings from substance abuse each year. Among patients who are alive on arrival to emergency departments, few die. It can be difficult to empathize with those who repeatedly and voluntarily overdose on various drugs. The emergency department becomes an important evaluation and triage center for these patients.

Overdose is properly treated in the emergency department by a medical team. Table 13–2 outlines the major medical complications and treatment approaches to various drug overdoses (The Medical Letter 1996). Because several drugs are slowly absorbed, the minimal time for observation of a suspected drug overdose should be 4 hours. Exact time of ingestion is often difficult to ascertain reliably. If there is good evidence that a specific drug was ingested, a call to the poison control center is suggested, and transfer to an emergency department is the next step. The first crucial step is to ensure the adequacy of airway, breathing, and circulation (ABC), which includes assessment of airway patency, respiratory rate, blood pressure, and pulse. Outside of the hospital, cardiopulmonary resuscitation (CPR) may be lifesaving. In the medical setting, every overdose patient with loss of consciousness or any patient with coma of unknown etiology should empirically receive 50 mg of dextrose 5% in water (D5W) and 0.4 mg of naloxone, which may need to be repeated. Prompt response supports evidence for hypoglycemia, opiate overdose, or alcohol overdose. In the case of Wernicke's encephalopathy, D5W should not be given first, because glucose can further suppress thiamine stores. Other basic measures in overdose include benzodiazepine treatment for status epilepticus and treatment of metabolic acidosis if present.

We emphasize general parameters of overdose elimination here (Table 13–3); the reader is referred elsewhere for technical information on elimination (Goldberg et al. 1986). *Gastric emptying* is appropriate only for drugs that are orally ingested. One absolute contraindication to gastric emptying is in cases of caustic ingestion. *Ipecac syrup* induces vomiting in approximately 30 minutes; to reduce the risk of aspiration it should be given only to patients who are awake and alert. It should be given even after spontaneous emesis because full gastric emptying may not have been accomplished. *Gastric lavage* entails flushing the upper gastrointestinal system with water. This technique is attempted only in patients who are unconscious and whose airway is secured by intubation. Placed in the stomach, *activated charcoal* serves as an absorbent to remove toxic substances and may reduce reabsorption of substances from the duodenum. When ingested substances are weak acids or bases, *forced diuresis* can be attempted in patients with functioning kidneys. *Hemodialysis* is generally a heroic measure to save a life and is most likely to be successful for drugs that are circulating in the plasma, minimally bound to tissue, and cleared poorly through the kidney. This technique has been especially valuable with alcohol, amphetamine, and aspirin overdose. *Hemoperfusion* is an extracorporeal blood-filtering technique like hemodialysis that uses a different type of membrane filtration. This technique has been especially useful in barbiturate overdose; however, it may lead to thrombocytopenia.

Intoxication

Most simple intoxication does not come to medical attention. Those cases that do present to the emergency department should be screened carefully for medical problems such as subdural hematomas, meningitis, human immunodeficiency virus (HIV) infection, or endocarditis with embolization. Support measures include interrupting substance absorption, providing a safe environment, decreasing sensory stimulation, and allowing the passage of time. A calm, nonthreatening manner should be employed, with clear communication and reality orientation. Attempts to reason with most intoxicated patients will not be fruitful; in cases of hallucinogen abuse, however, individuals can frequently be "talked down" from pathological intoxication. When concern exists that the intoxication will possibly lead to overdose, activism on the part of the clinician in calling for emergency medical services may be lifesaving. Involving family, AA sponsors, and members of support networks early in relapse can make it easier to achieve a stable situation faster.

Table 13–2.   Management of overdose

Drug	Major complications	Antidote/treatment	Potential lethal dose
Acetaminophen	Hepatotoxicity—peaks at 72–96 hours. Complete recovery generally in 4 days, but injury worse for alcoholics. Mortality: 1%–2%	N-acetylcysteine[a]	140 mg/kg
Alcohol	Respiratory depression	None	350–700 mg (serum)
Amphetamines	Seizures; avoid antipsychotics	None	20–25 mg/kg
Barbiturates	Respiratory depression	None	
Short-acting			>3 g
Long-acting			>6 g
Benzodiazepines	Sedation, respiratory depression, hypotension, coma	Flumazenil reverses effects (but may induce withdrawal in the dependent patient)	—
Carbon monoxide	Headaches, dizziness, weakness, nausea, vomiting, diminished visual acuity, tachycardia, tachypnea, ataxia, and seizures are all possible. Other manifestations include hemorrhages (cherry-red spots on the skin), metabolic acidosis, coma, and death.	Hyperbaric oxygen	—
Cocaine	Peak toxicity 60–90 minutes after use; systemic sympathomimesis and seizures, acidosis. Later, cardiopulmonary depression, perhaps pulmonary edema. Treatment of acidosis, seizures, and hypertension is imperative.	Naloxone (empirically)	—

Table 13–2. Management of overdose (continued)

Drug	Major complications	Antidote/treatment	Potential lethal dose
Hallucinogens	Ring-substituted amphetamines, or LSD/mescaline, may lead to rhabdomyolysis, hyperthermia, hyponatremia	Reduce temperature, dantrolene	—
Hydrocarbons	Gastrointestinal, respiratory, and CNS compromise	None	—
Hypnotics (non-BZD)	Delirium, EPS	None	Varies with tolerance
Inhalants	Cardiotoxicity, arrhythmias	Cardiac monitoring	—
Opioids	Miosis, respiratory depression, obtundation, pulmonary edema, delirium, death	Naloxone, nalmefene helpful	Varies with tolerance
Phencyclidine/ketamine	Hypertension, nystagmus, rhabdomyolysis	None; forced diuresis should not be attempted in cases of phencyclidine overdose with suspected rhabdomyolysis	—
Phenothiazines	Anticholinergism, EPS, cardiac effects	Phenothiazine overdose should be monitored for 48 hours for cardiac arrhythmia. Lidocaine may be necessary for treatment of cardiac arrhythmia, norepinephrine for hypotension, sodium bicarbonate for metabolic acidosis, and phenytoin for seizures	150 mg/kg
Salicylates	CNS, acidosis	None	500 mg/kg
TCAs	Cardiac effects, hypotension, anticholinergism	None	35 mg/kg

Note. — = unknown; BZD = benzodiazepine; CNS = central nervous system; LSD = lysergic acid diethylamide; EPS = extrapyramidal side effects; TCAs = tricyclic antidepressants. See Chapter 5 ("Definition, Presentation, and Diagnosis") for further discussion of overdose states.
aHeard KJ: Acetylcysteine for acetaminophen poisoning. *N Engl J Med* 359:285–292, 2008.

Table 13–3.   Overdose elimination methods

Drug	Ipecac syrup	Forced diuresis	Gastric lavage	Activated charcoal	Hemodialysis	Hemoperfusion
Acetaminophen	Yes	Yes (alkaline)	Yes	No	No	No
Alcohol	No	No	Yes	Yes	Yes	No
Amphetamines	Yes	Yes (acid)	Yes	Yes	Yes	
Barbiturates		Only for long-acting		Yes		Yes
Benzodiazepines	Yes	No	Yes	Repeated		
Carbon monoxide	No	No	No	No	No	No
Cocaine	No	No	No	No	No	No
Hydrocarbons	Yes	No	Yes			
Hypnotics (nonbenzodiazepine)	Yes	No	Yes	Yes		
Opioids						
Phencyclidine/ketamine	Only severe	Not in rhabdomyolysis (avoid in renal failure)	Only severe	Yes		
Phenothiazines	Yes		Yes	Yes		
Salicylates	Yes	Yes (alkaline)	Yes	Yes	Yes	
Tricyclic antidepressants				Repeated	No	No

Alcohol

There is no proven amethystic ("sobering-up") agent that can hasten the cessation of alcohol intoxication (not even strong black coffee or cold showers). There has been no shortage of experimental approaches to delaying absorption or decreasing metabolism and elimination, and both opiate antagonists (including naloxone) and central stimulants have also been studied as means to protect against dangerous effects of intoxication. The safe passage of time is currently the only effective measure to reverse acute intoxication.

Opioids

No specific measures are generally needed to treat opioid intoxication. If life-threatening overdose is suspected, prompt treatment with naloxone is necessary (see earlier discussion and Table 13–2). Accidental overdoses and deaths in the management of pain or use of methadone to treat opioid withdrawal have been increasingly reported. This is probably due to the narrow window between intoxication and overdose in oxycodone use. Physicians need more training in the proper use and dosing of opioids when these agents are required. It is beneficial that labeling changes have lowered recommended starting doses of opioids. Tolerance to opioids is reduced during abstinent periods, and overdose can occur when abuse of high doses of opioids is resumed.

Cocaine and Amphetamines

Individuals who abuse cocaine often self-medicate with central nervous system (CNS) depressants to counteract the dysphoric stimulant properties of the drug. For severe agitation, benzodiazepines such as diazepam or lorazepam may provide relief. If frank psychosis persists, low-dose haloperidol (2–5 mg) may be helpful, and the dose should be adjusted as necessary to control symptoms; however, haloperidol decreases the seizure threshold and thus should be used with caution. Monoamine oxidase inhibitors (MAOIs) should be avoided, given that they inhibit the degradation of cocaine and can produce a hypertensive crisis. In one of the few studies to examine outcome of cocaine dependence treatment, higher problem severity at admission and low treatment exposure were predictive of poorer long-term outcomes (Simpson et al. 2002).

Phencyclidine

The fundamental goal in treating the violence associated with phencyclidine (PCP) intoxication is to ensure the safety of all parties. When a patient becomes threatening, the strong physical presence of at least five people is needed for physical containment. Benzodiazepines such as diazepam are superior to antipsychotics during treatment of agitation, but antipsychotics such as haloperidol are better for PCP toxic psychosis. Enhancement of excretion is helpful, via gastric lavage (if orally administered) or via acidification of the urine (if systemic). For lasting problems, electroconvulsive therapy may be indicated.

Cannabis

Cannabis intoxication generally needs no formal treatment. The occasional severe anxiety attacks or acute paranoid episodes can be handled by reality orientation. In rare cases, severe anxiety may warrant treatment with a benzodiazepine. Low-dose haloperidol or olanzapine may be helpful for cannabis psychosis.

Hallucinogens

Patients experiencing hallucinogen intoxication can usually be "talked down" with reality orientation and reassurance. Benzodiazepines may help to provide sedation. Overdose, especially with 3,4-methylenedioxymethamphetamine (MDMA; Ecstasy), can lead to hyperpyrexia, dehydration, tachycardia, and even death, and should be treated in a medical setting.

Inhalants

Inhalant intoxication can vary in its presentation and need for active treatment. The main principle in treatment is protection of the individual from harm and from harming others. Symptoms are usually time-limited.

Withdrawal and Detoxification

Alcohol

Inpatient Versus Outpatient Setting

For treatment of alcohol SUDs, patients with delirium, low IQ, Wernicke's encephalopathy, trauma history, neurological symptoms, medical complications, psychopathology that requires medication, DTs or alcoholic seizures, or hallucinosis are probably best evaluated and treated in an inpatient setting. Polysubstance abuse, poor compliance, poor family support, lack of access to transportation, a chaotic or unstable home environment, or a home environment in which the patient is continually exposed to others with SUDs all predict poor outpatient detoxification success. Yet, outpatient detoxification can be appropriate: approximately 95% of patients have only mild to moderate withdrawal symptoms. Supportive care without pharmacological intervention is adequate for a significant number of these patients, and even when pharmacological intervention is needed, it can be given on an outpatient basis. Outpatient care reduces costs, allows the patient to continue to function in his or her environment, and provides time for the therapist to evaluate the patient's motivation for treatment.

Alcohol withdrawal implies at least physiological dependence, and careful attention to the risks of withdrawal is important. Unfortunately, in some centers, misguided practices remain in use that either are insufficiently precise or fail to achieve detoxification. For example, some practitioners provide medical inpatients with decreasing amounts of alcoholic beverages, such as beer, which is available in some hospital formularies. Other clinicians caring for nonpsychiatric or non-substance-related issues will choose not to detoxify—asserting that they are supporting the patient's lifestyle choice—and allow a steady ingestion of beer, even obtaining periodic tests of blood alcohol levels! The message and the methods in these situations are often inappropriate, indicating a failure to provide standard treatment and a lack of understanding of the serious nature of addictive disorders (Rosenbaum and McCarty 2002). At a minimum, individuals dependent on substances who are inpatient medical or surgical patients should receive appropriate detoxification, education, and referral for substance abuse treatment.

Pharmacological Versus Nonpharmacological Treatment

Most withdrawing alcohol users do not have major medical problems, but the best approach is conservative psychopharmacological management. Use of medication for the prevention of DTs or seizures is a top priority, not only to avoid discomfort and death but also to prevent acceleration of cognitive decline secondary to repeated uncontrolled withdrawal. Thus, pharmacological detoxification is warranted for those with significant signs of withdrawal, a clear history of severe daily dependence or high tolerance, codependence on other CNS depressants, or a history of DTs or seizures. Medical complications (e.g., infections, trauma, metabolic or hepatic disorders) indicate pharmacological treatment. Physical and subjective discomfort should be minimized. Pharmacological care enhances compliance and provides an alcohol-free interval that may help the patient commit to treatment. Negative countertransference of staff members can result in withholding of appropriate medication. There should be little to no concern that this treatment will make the alcoholic patient a benzodiazepine abuser. Nonpharmacological detoxification is for patients with mild symptoms or withdrawal history and mild to moderate dependence. Patients are housed for 3–4 days in a supportive, safe environment with rest and nutrition and detoxified without medication. This helps the patient to regulate and structure his or her life again. Close monitoring of patients for complications and adequate medical backup are needed for detoxification.

Pharmacological Withdrawal

For all patients withdrawing from alcohol, careful monitoring of vital signs, physical signs, and subjective symptoms must be done at least every 4 hours while the individual is awake (Table 13–4). Several objective rating scales and some subjective scales (e.g., Clinical Institute Withdrawal Assessment for Alcohol—Revised [CIWA-Ar; Sullivan et al. 1989] for those without general medical complications) are useful for monitoring the withdrawal state. Pharmacological detoxification essentially involves substituting alcohol with a drug that is cross-tolerant with alcohol and then slowly withdrawing the substitution drug from the body. For withdrawing patients with an altered mental status due to conditions other than alcohol (e.g., other substances, general medical or surgical conditions), detoxification remains a priority. Indeed, for those withdrawing from both opioids and alcohol, benzodiazepines might be given preferentially to methadone in order to substitute the alcohol while avoiding excessive sedation.

Benzodiazepine Treatment

Many agents benefit the withdrawal state somewhat, but with their agonist effect at the γ-aminobutyric acid (GABA) receptor, benzodiazepines are currently the best medications for alcohol detoxification. With adequate benzodiazepine coverage, complications of alcohol withdrawal are extremely rare. At usual

Table 13–4. Medical workup for alcohol withdrawal

Routine lab tests	CBC with differential, serum electrolytes, LFTs (including bilirubin), BUN, creatinine, fasting blood sugar, prothrombin time, cholesterol, triglycerides, calcium, magnesium, albumin, total protein, hepatitis B surface antigen, B_{12}, folate, stool guaiac, urinalysis, serum and urine toxic screens, CXR, ECG
Ancillary tests	EEG, CT, GI series, HIV, VDRL

Note. BUN = blood urea nitrogen; CBC = complete blood count; CT = computed tomography; CXR = chest X-ray; ECG = electrocardiogram; EEG = electroencephalogram; GI series = gastrointestinal radiography series; HIV = human immunodeficiency virus; LFTs = liver function tests; VDRL = venereal disease research laboratory.

doses, benzodiazepines produce little respiratory depression and provide a good margin of safety between effective dose and overdose. Chlordiazepoxide (Librium) and diazepam (Valium), the most commonly used benzodiazepines, are long acting. Once a sufficient dose has been given, they can be expected to "self-taper" without further dosing needed. With their lesser risk of accumulation and overdose, intermediate-half-life benzodiazepines such as lorazepam (Ativan) and oxazepam (Serax) are useful in elderly patients or in those with hepatic disease, delirium, dementia, or pulmonary disease. Lorazepam also has the advantages of primarily renal clearance and reliable intramuscular absorption. Table 13–5 presents treatment protocols for withdrawal. In all cases, thiamine (100 mg/day administered orally or intramuscularly), folic acid (1–3 mg/day), and multivitamins should also be added. When indicated, naltrexone or disulfiram can be added after a physical examination, an electrocardiogram, and blood work are obtained, in the absence of contraindications such as arrhythmias, heart disease, severe hepatic disease, esophageal varices, pregnancy, or a seizure disorder (discussed below), and after at least 72 hours have elapsed since last ingestion of alcohol.

Suppression of withdrawal symptoms does not substitute for systematic detoxification. A conservative 5- to 7-day regimen (see Table 13–5) promotes comfort, reduces complications, provides structure, and helps most patients cope cognitively and emotionally with the initial treatment. Uncomplicated detoxification of this length rarely occurs on an inpatient unit because of cost pressures, and inpatient alcohol detoxification is often condensed to 3 days. Outpatient detoxification for uncomplicated alcohol dependence can be accomplished within 4–5 days with chlordiazepoxide (25 mg four times a day,

Table 13–5. Benzodiazepine treatment for alcohol withdrawal

Outpatient	Chlordiazepoxide 25–50 mg po qid on first day, 20% decrease over 5 days, daily visits
Inpatient	1. Choose agent: diazepam or chlordiazepoxide—consider initial loading dose, then monitor objectively every 1–2 hours using vital signs or Clinical Institute Withdrawal Assessment (CIWA) scale (score greater than 9 being threshold) or both.
	2. Reassess for additional dose every 1–2 hours: chlordiazepoxide 25–50 mg (maximum 400 mg/24 hours), diazepam 5–10 mg (maximum 100 mg/24 hours), oxazepam 15–30 mg, or lorazepam 1 mg. Hold for sedation—sedation implies coverage is temporarily sufficient.
	3. Count total 24-hour dose needed for stabilization of signs.
	4. Total divided by 4 is amount to give four times a day.
	5. Taper daily total about 25% over 3 days—continue no more than 10 days.
	6. Use adjunctive treatments.
	7. Also administer thiamine 100 mg 4 times a day; folate 1 mg 4 times a day; multivitamin each day, $MgSO_4$ 1 g intramuscularly every 6 hours for 2 days if seizures occur (or carbamazepine or valproate).

decreasing to 0). Inpatient withdrawal from alcohol is accomplished with chlordiazepoxide (25–100 mg orally four times a day, with 25–50 mg every 2 hours as needed [prn] for positive withdrawal signs). Doses can be held if the patient appears intoxicated. Both regimens should include thiamine (50–100 mg/day orally or intramuscularly), folate (1–3 mg/day) and multivitamins. Naltrexone is usually added 5 days after detoxification.

Adjuncts to Benzodiazepines

Seizure protection. Consideration of patients at imminent risk of withdrawal seizures or DTs should be a part of all detoxification strategies. Antiepileptic drugs are not routinely prescribed prophylactically unless the patient has a history of a seizure disorder. Those who have experienced seizures during withdrawal do not always receive anticonvulsant medications. Gabapentin, which is renally excreted and lacks significant drug–drug interactions, cognitive effects, and abuse potential, is an ideal medication for patients with a history of seizures during withdrawal. Phenytoin was previously used for this purpose, and valproate may be used as well. Magnesium sulfate (1 g four times a day for 2 days) is also useful.

Autonomic nervous system signs. Both beta-blockers (e.g., propranolol) and alpha-blockers (e.g., clonidine) may alleviate autonomic nervous system signs and symptoms that occur during withdrawal. For propranolol, the usual dosage is 10 mg every 6 hours as needed; for clonidine, it is 0.5 mg two to three times a day as needed.

Psychotic features. Antipsychotics are helpful if the withdrawal syndrome includes delirium, delusions, or hallucinations. Haloperidol 0.5–2.0 mg can be administered intramuscularly every 2 hours.

Other Central Nervous System Depressants

Withdrawal from benzodiazepines, barbiturates, or other depressants often requires pharmacological detoxification. This is true for benzodiazepines used in high doses for short periods or low to medium dosages for long periods of time (i.e., months, years). Conservative treatment requires a slow withdrawal over many days or weeks. Withdrawal from benzodiazepines can generally be accomplished with chlordiazepoxide or diazepam (long half-life). A standard benzodiazepine detoxification regimen is outlined in Table 13–6. If the abuse history is unreliable or difficult to ascertain, a pentobarbital challenge test can be used to find a starting dose (Table 13–7). Benzodiazepine detoxification is best done on an inpatient unit, except for those patients who have been on a low dose for a very long time. Outpatient detoxification for the chronic low-dose benzodiazepine user occurs over 6–12 weeks of gradual reduction, dur-

Table 13–6. Benzodiazepine detoxification

1. Establish usual maintenance dose by history or pentobarbital tolerance test (Table 13–7).
2. Divide maintenance dose into equivalent as-needed doses of diazepam and administer first 2 days.
3. Decrease diazepam 10% each day thereafter.
4. Administer diazepam 5 mg every 6 hours, as needed, for signs of increased withdrawal.
5. When diazepam dose approaches 10% of original, reduce dose slowly over 3–4 days, then discontinue.

Table 13–7.   Pentobarbital challenge test: clinical response to 200 mg test dose of pentobarbital

Patient condition after test dose	Degree of tolerance	Estimated 24-hour pentobarbital requirement (mg)
Asleep but arousable	None or minimal	None
Drowsy; slurred speech; ataxia, marked intoxication	Definite but mild	400–600
Comfortable; fine lateral nystagmus only	Marked	600–1,000
No signs of effect; abstinence signs persist	Extreme	1,000–1,200 or more: In this case, give 100 mg every 2 hours (to a maximum of 500 mg) until mild intoxication is produced. Multiply the amount that produced mild intoxication by 4 to give the estimated 24-hour dose of pentobarbital, and convert to phenobarbital equivalents (100 mg of pentobarbital = 30 mg of phenobarbital). Give that phenobarbital dose for 2 days and then taper by 30 mg/day or 10% per day, whichever is less

Note.   For benzodiazepine discontinuation, assess clinical response 1 hour after 200 mg test dose of pentobarbital.

ing which time added support and education are helpful. The option of a prn dose to avoid feeling trapped is fine. The worst symptoms occur at the lowest doses and in the first week without any medication. All parties should be prepared: the stress of that week may make it seem like a year.

After detoxification, patients should be referred to AA, Narcotics Anonymous, or Al-Anon. For those who originally presented with anxiety, rebound can be expected. Nonbenzodiazepine alternatives for anxiety include cognitive-behavioral therapy, exercise, relaxation, and psychotherapy. One in eight patients will develop severe postdetoxification anxiety requiring treatment with medications and/or cognitive-behavioral therapy.

Many CNS depressants (e.g., glutethimide [Doriden]), are abused episodically and do not require formal detoxification. For barbiturate or methaqualone abuse, detoxification is necessary. Barbiturate detoxification can be accomplished with a long-acting benzodiazepine or a long-acting barbiturate, such as phenobarbital.

In some cases, there is a need to substitute one CNS depressant for another. Most such "cross-tapers" occur over 3 weeks with the use of clonazepam. In week 1, the patient takes clonazepam 0.5 mg at bedtime and the previously used drug on a prn basis. In week 2, the previously used drug is discontinued. In week 3, the clonazepam dose is reduced to 0. This regimen requires inpatient admission for patients with nonbenzodiazepine abuse, those with polysubstance abuse, or those who have failed to respond to outpatient treatment. The pentobarbital tolerance test should be used to set the initial dose when a patient's dosage of use is unknown. Alprazolam (Xanax) is uniquely less amenable to drug substitution. Breakthrough seizures have been reported despite adequate coverage with chlordiazepoxide. Alprazolam detoxification should include an estimation of daily use and a slow withdrawal over a period of several weeks. Clonazepam has also been successfully used in alprazolam detoxification.

Opioids

Standard Detoxification Protocol: Methadone

Opioid detoxification may be needed to interrupt an opioid-related SUD. These patients rarely seek treatment; when they do come in voluntarily, it is often a consequence of an interrupted supply, an overdose, or a failed attempt at self-detoxification. Methadone detoxification can be difficult because of the drug's long half-life and the typically chronic use.

Until the advent of buprenorphine, the most common detoxification approach was to substitute and then taper a long-acting opioid (usually an equivalent dose of methadone). For most heroin addicts, 20 mg methadone is adequate as an initial dose (30 mg is the maximum initial dose in federally licensed facilities), and the patient should be reevaluated every 2–4 hours to determine whether additional doses are necessary. Once a stable dose is achieved, methadone should be decreased over 4–14 days, usually by 5 mg/day. Published ratios of pure drug to methadone can help in determining an initial dose, but the clinician should be aware that there is uncertainty as to the exact ratios. Table 13–8 provides dose equivalents among opioids.

Another approach is to slowly taper the abused drug over time. This is untenable for illicit drugs, but codeine, for example, could be detoxified in this way. The estimated amount used daily is mixed with 30 mg cherry syrup and given every day over 7–10 days, with the amount of drug decreased daily. A low dose (25–50 mg) of thioridazine (Mellaril) concentrate can be added to reduce subjective discomfort.

Table 13–8. Approximate dose equivalents for opioids

Drug[a]	Oral dose (mg)	Parenteral dose
Morphine	30	10 mg
Methadone	10–20	N/A
Meperidine	300	75 mg
Codeine	200	100–120 mg
Fentanyl	N/A	100 µg
Hydrocodone (Vicodin)	30–45	N/A
Hydromorphone (Dilaudid)	8	2 mg
Oxycodone (Oxycontin)	20–30	10–15 mg
Propoxyphene (Darvon, Darvocet)	130	130
Oxymorphone (Opana, Opana ER, Opana IV)	10	1 mg

Note.   N/A = not available.
[a]Based on standard 10 mg intravenous morphine.

Source.   Adapted from National Cancer Institute (http://www.cancer.gov/cancertopics/pdq/supportivecare/pain/HealthProfessional/Table3; accessed March 5, 2009).

Clonidine

Clonidine is an α_2 agonist that has been shown to effectively suppress signs and symptoms of autonomic sympathetic activation during withdrawal. (It has been less successful in decreasing the subjective discomfort of withdrawal.) Clonidine detoxification is most successful in individuals with mild dependence, high motivation, and inpatient status. Detoxification usually takes 10–14 days. On the first day of treatment, oral clonidine is begun at a dosage of 0.1–0.3 mg three times a day (maximum 1.2 mg/day); on the third day, the dosage is increased to 0.4–0.7 mg three times a day, and this dosage is maintained for the rest of the detoxification period. In appropriate patients, naltrexone can be started during clonidine detoxification, as described in Table 13–9 (Simpson et al. 2002). The major side effects of clonidine are hypotension and sedation. Vital signs should be monitored carefully for patients taking clonidine. Clonidine detoxification may be conducted on an outpatient basis with highly motivated patients (O'Connor et al. 1995). Lofexidine, a centrally acting α_2 agonist, may be comparable to clonidine but is not yet approved by the U.S. Food and Drug Administration for this purpose.

Buprenorphine

Since its introduction, buprenorphine has grown in popularity as an agent to use in the initial care of persons who are opioid dependent. Because it blocks withdrawal, it is useful for detoxification from other opioids. Most patients can be stabilized on a low dose of sublingual buprenorphine (e.g., 8 mg/day), and if total detoxification is the goal, the dose can be reduced at 2 mg decrements without producing significant withdrawal symptoms. In order to prevent precipitated withdrawal, use of buprenorphine in this fashion must not begin until the end of intoxication and the onset of withdrawal. Although prescribing buprenorphine in acute detoxification is an approved practice (Substance Abuse and Mental Health Services Administration 2004), buprenorphine's efficacy compared with methadone or clonidine is unknown. Detoxification using buprenorphine is only one step in the process, and it should be followed by attention to long-term relapse prevention.

Rapid and Ultrarapid Detoxification Approaches

Rapid and ultrarapid detoxification approaches use opioid antagonists and adjuncts such as clonidine, sedation, and even general anesthesia; they are

Table 13–9.   Ambulatory opioid detoxification medication protocols

| 9-day protocol | 9-day clonidine detoxification | | | |
	Day 1	Days 2, 3, 4	Days 5, 6, 7	Days 8, 9
Clonidine	0.1–0.2 mg; maximum dose: 1 mg	0.1–0.2 mg po four times a day as needed; maximum dose: 1.2 mg	Taper to 0	0
Naltrexone				Day 8: 25 mg; day 9: 50 mg

| 5-day protocol | 5-day clonidine detoxification ending with induction of naltrexone 50 mg/day | | |
	Days 1, 2	Days 3, 4, 5	
Clonidine	Preload 0.2–0.4 mg po three times a day; maximum dose: 1.2 mg	Taper to 0	
Oxazepam	Preload 30–60 mg	0	
Naltrexone	Day 1: 12.5 mg; day 2: 25 mg	50 mg po each day	

performed at few institutions. The goal is to detoxify in a manner so as to avoid the need for long-term methadone maintenance. These methods are used for patients in transition to antagonist therapy (e.g., with naltrexone). Unfortunately, ultrarapid detoxification has the increased risks of anesthesia, is often done without rehabilitation, and is expensive. The use of subcutaneous naltrexone pellets poses risks of serious complications such as pulmonary edema, variceal rupture, or death (Hamilton et al. 2002).

Detoxification Adjuncts

Detoxification with clonidine as an adjunct treatment should take 5–6 days; it is unlikely to be helpful beyond 14 days. Clonidine can be administered transdermally via a patch. Its use should be avoided at night. Benzodiazepines are helpful for insomnia. At low dosages (2–4 mg/day), buprenorphine is useful as a partial agonist because it blocks withdrawal; however, at larger doses it decreases respiratory drive. Other drugs that can be helpful adjuncts during opioid withdrawal include dicyclomine (Bentyl) for gastrointestinal pain, nonsteroidal anti-inflammatory drugs for myalgias, and antiemetics.

Maintenance and Relapse Prevention

Adult long-term users of opioids often become trapped in a cycle of repeated unsuccessful detoxifications. To help break this cycle, clinicians should encourage those who meet criteria to try long-term methadone maintenance or office-based buprenorphine treatment. For many with chronic opioid dependence, substitution and maintenance is the treatment of choice and should more often be recommended. Opioid agonist substitution is the key to long-term recovery. Methadone is the standard, but buprenorphine is also effective in the attempt to interrupt the addictive lifestyle, promote stability and employment, decrease intravenous drug use and its attendant risk of hepatitis B or HIV, and reduce criminal activity (Schwartz et al. 2006). Methadone is a long-acting (half-life: 24–36 hours), cross-tolerant opioid that mutes extreme fluctuation in serum opioid levels and blunts euphoric response to heroin. Given once daily, methadone provides a structure for rehabilitation. Starting dosages are usually 20–40 mg/day, depending on degree of dependence, and may require an increase to 120 mg/day. Maintenance dosages of 70 mg/day and above lead to fewer relapses. Narcotics Anonymous–oriented rehabilitation programs or therapeutic communities may exclude patients on methadone. Debate surrounds the substitution model, but the positive effects of methadone are vital to a subset of patients.

A large number of patients have successfully interrupted their drug-using lifestyles using methadone maintenance. Unfortunately, only 20%–25% of addicted individuals receive this treatment. It is primarily indicated for the hard-core addict and for patients who are HIV positive, who are pregnant, or who have a history of legal problems. Methadone maintenance is contraindicated for anyone who is younger than 16 years, who is to be jailed within 30–45 days, or who has a history of abusing the medicine. Many addicted patients have compromised liver function due to alcohol abuse or hepatitis, and methadone use may be contraindicated for patients with severe liver damage. Many individuals remain on methadone for several years. When indicated, withdrawal should be accomplished slowly to minimize discomfort; this is often a protracted affair. Generally, the medication should not be decreased more than 10% per week. Below 10–20 mg of methadone, subjective symptoms of withdrawal may intensify and necessitate a further decrease in the rate of withdrawal to 3% per week. Iatrogenic withdrawal often leads to relapse. It is useful to remember the half-lives of the opioids: morphine sulfate, 2–3 hours; methadone, 15–25 hours.

Antagonist Maintenance

Naltrexone is an opioid antagonist (see discussion below) that when used regularly leads to gradual extinction of drug-seeking behavior. Its efficacy is less than that of methadone or buprenorphine. For opioid relapse prevention, naltrexone is usually given at a dosage of 25–50 mg/day for the first 5–10 days, which is gradually increased to 50–100 mg daily or three times weekly. High refusal and dropout rates limit this agent's use to highly motivated individuals with a good prognosis who are likely to do well in a variety of treatment options and with whom there is a good treatment alliance. Naltrexone can be used long-term in the outpatient setting. It is valuable in abstinence-oriented treatment. When taken within 7 days of opioid use, naltrexone may induce withdrawal; the clinician should determine the risk of this situation. With the exception of clonidine-assisted protocols of induction (see Table 13–9), naltrexone should not be given to individuals who may be dependent on opioids.

Cocaine, Cannabis, Hallucinogens, and Inhalants

No specific pharmacological detoxification protocols are available for cocaine, cannabis, hallucinogens, or inhalants. General supportive measures are usually adequate; acupuncture may even be helpful for cocaine detoxification. Benzodiazepines may alleviate discomfort in the cocaine-withdrawing patient, but they pose the potential for abuse. Other medications that may relieve the symptoms of cocaine abstinence include the tricyclic antidepressant desipramine (which is superior to lithium for this indication), other antidepressants, carbamazepine, and perhaps buprenorphine when opioids have been used as well as cocaine. Suicide precautions should be taken with such patients when they are depressed or psychotic. Modafinil is used experimentally in some centers to ease withdrawal.

For inhalant-induced psychosis, carbamazepine has efficacy comparable to that of haloperidol but without extrapyramidal side effects or lowering of the seizure threshold (Hernandez-Avila et al. 1998).

Individuals in the dangerous amphetamine-like state caused by ring-substituted amphetamine hallucinogens (MDMA, 3,4-methylenedioxyamphetamine [MDA]) should be closely monitored; supportive treatment, including hydration and monitoring for hyperpyrexia, and perhaps dantrolene, should be provided. The sympathomimetic state produced by lysergic acid diethylamide (LSD) and mescaline also requires support. Patients experiencing anxiety due to use of LSD and mescaline require reassurance and reorientation. Usually restraint can be avoided. For the psychological sequelae of hallucinogens, benzodiazepines are superior to first-generation antipsychotics.

Nicotine

There is no specific protocol for withdrawal from nicotine per se, but numerous modalities are available to assist in smoking cessation and maintenance of abstinence, such as a nicotine patch with gradual reductions. For detailed information and further resources, the clinician should consult the most recent Surgeon General's report (U.S. Department of Health and Human Services 2000) or the Centers for Disease Control and Prevention (CDC) guidelines, which are periodically revised (Fiore et al. 2008). Many guidelines for smoking cessation have been published (American Psychiatric Association 1996). It is unnecessary for inpatient substance use programs to defer smoking cessation treatment until after discharge—such treatment actually improves long-term sobriety rates from alcohol and other drugs as well as short-term nicotine quit rates, although the success rate of nicotine cessation is not necessarily improved over the long term (Prochaska et al. 2004).

Relapse, unfortunately, is common, although patients who are determined to stop eventually do so, especially when they seek out effective help; even those who attempt quitting without assistance are ultimately successful more often than not. The primary care provider's assistance is essential. Compliance is greater with the nicotine patch than with nicotine chewing gum. Bupropion SR (sustained release) is also helpful. Scheduled dosing may be better than prn dosing. A nasal spray and an inhaler are also available but are not considered first-line treatments. Other than bupropion, which has demonstrated benefit, other antidepressants and clonidine may be helpful. A new medication, varenicline, is also being prescribed. It too has many pros and cons, which are discussed in Chapter 12 ("Treatment Modalities").

Motivation to change is a key aspect of successful smoking cessation. Selecting the most appropriate treatment requires a thorough history of the factors that led to smoking. The individual's self-efficacy and sense that he or she "can do it" greatly influences the potential for success. Patient motivation is also the basis for the success of interventions such as education, contingency management, and brief physician advice. Motivation and self-efficacy should be assessed and addressed at every step.

Nonpharmacological methods that have been studied in smoking cessation include self-help, clinical interventions (both minimal and intensive), behavioral treatment (including cue exposure and aversive strategies such as rapid smoking), nicotine fading, motivational rewards, social support, hypnosis, and acupuncture.

Although there is abundant evidence of the effectiveness of nicotine replacement via gum or patch, it should be noted that the CDC guidelines (Fiore et al. 2008) emphasize the need to pair these strategies with some degree of psychosocial treatment because the combination increases the likelihood of success.

Polysubstance Use

Detoxification

Polysubstance use makes detoxification more difficult. Concurrent withdrawal from multiple substances confuses the clinical picture. For detoxification from both CNS depressants and opioids, detoxification of the former is the priority, given the life-threatening nature of CNS depressant withdrawal and the length of opiate detoxification. Also, combining benzodiazepines and methadone risks overdose and requires close patient monitoring and dose adjustments as needed. Simultaneous detoxification from drugs of different classes can greatly increase physical or psychological discomfort and lead to higher elopement or relapse (Eric et al. 2005).

Integration of Treatment Approaches

Polysubstance abuse has been inadequately addressed by the treatment system. Drug and alcohol programs are often separately funded. Alcohol counselors may lack the training or interest to treat polysubstance abuse. Until recently, AA groups had difficulty integrating younger individuals with polysubstance abuse into their membership. Unfortunately, an attitude of "my addiction is better than your addiction" can develop. In clinical settings, such attitudes must be confronted with education and greater tolerance of social differences among patients. The exclusively alcoholic middle-aged white male, once common in treatment facilities, is now outnumbered by a younger, polysubstance-addicted, and more heterogeneous population (including larger numbers of women) with additional psychiatric problems.

Special Issues in Treatment

Mentally Ill, Chemically Abusing Patients

Most psychiatric patients have more than one psychiatric diagnosis; the most frequent comorbid diagnoses are SUDs. Every patient with an SUD needs a careful psychiatric assessment and treatment plan. Conversely, a thorough substance use history is an essential part of all psychiatric interviews. Interactions between SUDs and other psychiatric diagnoses must be integrated into treatment planning. SUDs may be comorbid with disorders of mood, anxiety, and personality as well as with organic disorders, schizophrenia, or anorexia nervosa. SUDs can mask, mimic, or result from a wide variety of psychiatric and medical disorders. The psychiatrist provides an understanding of the SUD in relation to other psychiatric illness and determines the course of action at the most appropriate level, be it psychosocial or medical. Once its comorbidity is established, a co-occurring psychiatric condition such as depression should be treated concurrently with the substance use (Ries and Comtois 1997).

Longitudinal, adoption, epidemiological, and family studies have not definitively settled old questions as to the cause, effect, or coexistent relationship between psychopathology and addictive behavior. Most studies support the idea that the inherited predisposition to addiction is independent of other psychiatric disorders. The trait of addiction may be primary to psychiatric illness, may develop as a way of coping with other problems, or may coexist with other psychiatric disorders. Treatment planning for substance-abusing patients with mental illness depends on flexibility and a broad understanding of psychiatry, as well as an understanding of alcohol and drug abuse.

Dual-Diagnosis Patients

Complex interactions between psychopathology and addictions are hard to separate clinically because of overlapping signs and symptoms resulting from intoxication, withdrawal, mixed drug reactions, adverse drug responses, medical conditions, and the organic and psychosocial effects of substance use on affective state, anxiety, or personality. The addition of other Axis I, II, and III disorders complicates diagnoses and makes addiction treatment more difficult. Also, treatment of addictions in patients with psychiatric illness is made complicated by risk of violence toward self or others associated with anxiety; irritation, anger, impulsivity, and poor reality testing in intoxication or withdrawal; and aggressivity on use of cocaine, hallucinogens, PCP, or alcohol.

Personnel in the mental health field and the substance abuse field should have the rudimentary knowledge to screen patients properly and to develop a treatment plan that adequately addresses the patients' needs. Model programs have been developed around the country to integrate psychiatric and substance abuse treatment. However, the dual-diagnosis patient often falls through the cracks of the treatment system. Severe psychiatric disorders often preclude full treatment in substance abuse clinics or self-help groups. Confrontational techniques and self-exposure, as used in some substance abuse programs, may exacerbate psychiatric symptoms. Special AA and Narcotics

Anonymous groups are being formed for dual-diagnosis or "double trouble" patients. High-psychiatric-severity patients benefit significantly from additional professional psychiatric therapy. Some patients, especially patients with frank psychosis or suicidal ideation, require primary psychiatric settings (e.g., day hospital or inpatient setting). However, treatment for primary psychiatric disorders should not preclude addressing substance abuse issues. Attendance at AA or Narcotics Anonymous meetings should be arranged, if possible. An addiction psychiatrist should be available to psychiatric facilities with a high number of dual-diagnosis patients. The addiction psychiatrist may be best used as part of a multidisciplinary team approach.

A discussion of treatment of dual-diagnosis patients would not be complete without the recognition of some of the pressing social needs of these patients. Often, patients with SUDs have alienated family, friends, and treatment personnel. The need for adequate housing, health, and follow-up is imperative. Residential facilities are needed to ease the transition of these patients into society. Coordination of the various agencies is necessary. Talbott (1981) discussed the case management approach extensively. There is evidence that integrated ("wraparound") care helps. However, substance abuse facilities often refuse admission to psychiatric patients, and psychiatric facilities may refuse patients with a history of substance abuse.

Psychiatric patients who abuse drugs pose interesting questions when it comes to choosing psychopharmacological treatment with other abusable medications. For example, patients with attention-deficit/hyperactivity disorder (ADHD) who abuse cocaine are at high risk for treatment failure or dropout. Notwithstanding plausible controversy over the use of stimulants in persons with substance abuse disorders, use of sustained-release methylphenidate (Ritalin) may help these patients.

Rehabilitation

The rehabilitation model, pioneered in the treatment of substance abuse, has become an important model for a variety of categories of psychiatric illness. It combines self-help, counseling, education, relapse prevention, group treatment, a warm supportive environment, and emphasis on a medical model geared to reducing stigma and blame. Most treatment units are highly structured, insist on an abstinence goal, and use lectures, films, and discussion groups as part of a complete cognitive and educational program. Patients are frequently converted into active 12-Step members and are encouraged to continue in aftercare.

A highly skilled professional team with available consultation is needed to integrate counseling; cognitive and behavioral treatment; relapse prevention strategies; interpersonal, family, and group therapy; applied or brief psychodynamically oriented psychotherapy; social network approaches; education; and occupational and recreational therapy. Inpatient programs previously included 5–7 days for detoxification and 3–6 weeks for rehabilitation, but now parts of rehabilitation are often done in halfway houses in outpatient settings, and hospital stays of 3–12 days are more common. Longer stays are indicated for adolescents and for patients with greater severity of illness, dual diagnoses, or severe medical problems.

The rehabilitation model emphasizes providing opportunities for patients to practice social skills, gain control over impulses, and use the highly structured program as an auxiliary superego, and it encourages self-honesty and expression of feelings. The program promotes the use of higher-level defenses (e.g., intellectualization) and actively confronts more primitive defenses (e.g., denial, splitting, and projection), especially when these defenses are used in regard to the issue of abstinence (Frances and Alexopoulos 1982).

Rehabilitation can take place in freestanding rehabilitation programs, mental illness/chemical abuse (MICA) units, general hospitals, inpatient programs, organized outpatient day and evening hospitals, therapeutic communities, and halfway houses. Addiction day treatment programs, which utilize many of the same techniques employed in inpatient treatment programs, are staffed by interdisciplinary teams that develop individualized treatment plans. Organized outpatient alcohol programs may provide a range of treatment modalities of varying intensity. These programs are less restrictive than and provide an alternative to hospitalization and may be useful as part of an aftercare program.

Aftercare

On patient discharge from an inpatient or organized outpatient program, aftercare must be part of the care plan. Referral to a 12-Step program often complements other treatment, although self-help may suffice for some faithfully attending people. We recommend at least 2 years of follow-up after start of abstinence.

Key Points

- A therapeutic alliance will enhance any treatment approach.
- Addiction must be diagnosed and is a treatable disease.
- Frequently addicted patients have comorbid medical and psychiatric problems that must be treated in synchrony.
- Cognitive and pharmacological approaches are safe and effective and often can be combined.
- Treatment should take on the special needs related to gender, age, cultural, and religious beliefs, and mental health and addiction treatment must be seamless and integrated.

References

American Psychiatric Association: Practice guideline for the treatment of patients with nicotine dependence. Am J Psychiatry 153 (10 suppl):1–31, 1996

Anton RF, O'Malley SS, Ciraulo DA, et al: Combined pharmacotherapies and behavioral interventions for alcohol dependence: the COMBINE study: a randomized controlled trial. JAMA 295:2003–2017, 2006

Armour D, Polich J, Stambul H: Alcoholism and Treatment. New York, Wiley, 1978

Compton WM, Thomas YF, Stinson FS, et al: Prevalence, correlates, disability, and comorbidity of DSM-IV drug abuse and dependence in the United States: results from the national epidemiologic survey on alcohol and related conditions. Arch Gen Psychiatry 64:566–576, 2007

Eric D, Collins, Herbert D, et al: Anesthesia-assisted vs buprenorphine- or clonidine-assisted heroin detoxification and naltrexone induction: a randomized trial. JAMA 294:903–913, 2005

Fiore MC, Jaén CR, Baker TB, et al: Treating Tobacco Use and Dependence: 2008 Update. Clinical Practice Guideline. Rockville, MD, U.S. Department of Health and Human Services, 2008

Frances RJ, Alexopoulos GS: The inpatient treatment of the alcoholic patient. Psychiatric Ann 12:386–391, 1982

Goldberg MJ, Spector R, Park GD, et al: An approach to the management of the poisoned patient. Arch Intern Med 146:1381–1385, 1986

Hamilton RJ, Olmedo RE, Shah S, et al: Complications of ultrarapid opioid detoxification with subcutaneous naltrexone pellets. Acad Emerg Med 9:63–68, 2002

Heard KJ: Acetylcysteine for acetaminophen poisoning. N Engl J Med 359:285–292, 2008

Hernandez-Avila CA, Ortega-Soto HA, Jasso A, et al: Treatment of inhalant-induced psychotic disorder with carbamazepine versus haloperidol. Psychiatr Serv 49:812–815, 1998

Kessler RC, Aguilar-Gaxiola S, Berglund PA, et al: Patterns and predictors of treatment seeking after onset of a substance use disorder. Arch Gen Psychiatry 58:1065–1071, 2001

Marlatt GA, Gordon JR: Relapse Prevention: Maintenance Strategies in the Treatment of Addictive Behaviors. New York, Guilford, 1985

McLellan AT, Grissom GR, Zanis D, et al: Problem-service matching in addiction treatment: a prospective study in 4 programs. Arch Gen Psychiatry 54:730–735, 1997

Mee-Lee D, Shulman GR, Fishman M, et al: ASAM PPC-2R: American Society of Addiction Medicine Patient Placement Criteria for the Treatment of Substance-Related Disorders, 2nd Edition—Revised. Chevy Chase, MD, American Academy of Addiction Medicine, 2001

O'Connor PG, Waugh ME, Carrol KM, et al: Primary care-based ambulatory opioid detoxification: the results of a clinical trial. J Gen Intern Med 10:255–260, 1995

Prochaska JJ, Delucci K, Hall SM, et al: A meta-analysis of smoking cessation interventions with individuals in substance abuse treatment or recovery. J Consult Clin Psychol 72:1144–1156, 2004

Ries RK, Comtois KA: Illness severity and treatment services for dually diagnosed severely mentally ill outpatients. Schizophr Bull 23:239–246, 1997

Ritsher JB, Moos RH, Finney JW: Relationship of treatment orientation and continuing care to remission among substance abuse patients. Psychiatr Serv 53:595–601, 2002

Rosenbaum M, McCarty T: Alcohol prescription by surgeons in the prevention and treatment of delirium tremens: historic and current practice. Gen Hosp Psychiatry 24:257–259, 2002

Schwartz RP, Highfield DA, Jaffe JH, et al: A randomized controlled trial of interim methadone maintenance. Arch Gen Psychiatry 63:102–109, 2006

Simpson DD, Joe GW, Broome KM: A national 5-year follow-up of treatment outcomes for cocaine dependence. Arch Gen Psychiatry 59:538–544, 2002

Substance Abuse and Mental Health Services Administration, Center for Substance Abuse Treatment: Clinical Guidelines for the Use of Buprenorphine in the Treatment of Opioid Addiction. Treatment Improvement Protocol (TIP) Series 40; Publ No SMA 04-3939. Rockville, MD, U.S. Department of Health and Human Services, 2004

Sullivan JT, Sykora K, Schneiderman J, et al: Assessment of alcohol withdrawal: the revised Clinical Institute Withdrawal Assessment for Alcohol scale (CIWA-Ar). Br J Addict 84:1353–1357, 1989

Talbott J (ed): The Chronic Mentally Ill: Treatment, Programs, Systems. New York, Human Sciences Press, 1981

The Medical Letter: Acute reactions to drugs of abuse. Med Lett Drugs Ther 38:43–46, 1996

U.S. Department of Health and Human Services: Reducing Tobacco Use: A Report of the Surgeon General. Atlanta, GA, Centers for Disease Control and Prevention, National Center for Chronic Disease Prevention and Health Promotion, Office on Smoking and Health, 2000

14

Public Health Issues

In this chapter, three segments of societal approaches to substance use are reviewed: workplace, public sector clinical, and public policy on prevention and control.

The Workplace

The workplace is an important setting for surveillance and intervention of substance use disorders (SUDs). Most adults with an SUD are employed, and an estimated 29% of all full-time workers engage in binge drinking and 8% in heavy drinking; 8% have used drugs in the past month (Merrick et al. 2007). Among employed adults, the highest rates of current drug use and heavy drinking are reported by white non-Hispanic males 18–25 years old with less than a high school education (Merrick et al. 2007). These are often users who have changed jobs frequently.

Based on 2002 estimates, the same proportion applies to the nation's 51.1 million adult binge drinkers and the 15.2 million adult heavy drinkers (Substance Abuse and Mental Health Services Administration 2007). A 1997 study of workplace alcohol use indicated that 7.6% of full-time employees are heavy drinkers (defined as 5 or more drinks on 5 or more days in the month prior to survey), and that 33% of those were also using illicit drugs (Merrick et al. 2007).

Alcohol and drug substances weigh heavily on American business. For illicit drugs, the overall societal cost of drug abuse in 1998 was $143.4 billion. Lost productivity accounted for around $100 billion of that figure (Office of National Drug Control Policy 2001). The best estimate for the cost of alcohol is much higher, at $185 billion, with lost productivity accounting for around $130 billion (National Institute on Alcohol Abuse and Alcoholism 2001). Drinking at work, problem drinking, and frequency of "getting drunk" in the prior 30 days are associated with frequency of absenteeism, arriving late to work and/or leaving early, doing poor work, doing less work, and arguing with coworkers, described as "presenteeism" (National Institute on Alcohol Abuse and Alcoholism 1999).

Increasingly since the 1980s, the military, a large number of major corporations, and insurance carriers have recognized the value of early identification and evaluation of chemical dependency problems and have offered their chemically dependent employees opportunities for treatment and assistance, including employee assistance programs (EAPs) or general fitness and wellness programs. The hidden benefits of rehabilitation programs are not lost on administrators concerned with cost-effectiveness. In addition to retaining valuable employees, the corporations find that these programs reduce union pressure that could occur from firing employees whose job performances do not improve because they fail to follow through with treatment. Unions have also recognized the valuable health benefits side of EAPs as a way of improving labor-management relations.

Case-Finding at the Workplace

In our culture, the greatest pressure that leads individuals with SUDs to accept treatment occurs in the workplace. Usually, people with SUDs do not seek help until a crisis has occurred somewhere in their lives. Frequently, people will not seek treatment, even though they may have marital, medical, or other problems, until their jobs are threatened. Fellow employees and managers may be overprotective of a troubled employee and wait until a crisis occurs that leads to firing. It is helpful to train supervisors that early recognition of job performance problems and referral to an EAP for evaluation can result in protection of jobs as well as improved health. Individuals with SUDs who still have jobs and marriages intact have the best prognosis.

The Employee Assistance Program Model

EAPs have evolved during the past few decades. Previously, the typical EAP was staffed by "recovering," nonclinical personnel and the office had little or no visibility with senior leadership, had a less-than-ideal relationship with external mental health and substance abuse practitioners, and was reactive rather than proactive. Now they are more and more proactive, with "stress debriefing" after critical incidents, and have workplace violence teams as well. Unfortunately, human resources managers restrict substance abuse service coverage to a great extent.

Most EAPs have both voluntary and mandatory portals of entry. Once workers see the program is successful for others, many volunteer for treatment. The EAP basically provides the employee with another opportunity to improve work performance with the addition of treatment. Information obtained during the process is not shared with the supervisor and is kept confidential. Ultimate job action depends on job performance rather than on the recommendation of either the EAP counselor or the treatment resource. Confidentiality is essential to any successful EAP. EAP enrollment rose from 27.2 million individuals in 1993 to 80.2 million in 2002 (Open Minds 2002). The "success rate" of the EAP has been cited to be 70% (Blum et al. 1992), although outcome measures require further refinement.

Job Impairment

Employees may experience problems related to either the use of substances on the job or the effects of chronic abuse that takes place after work hours. Disability may include medical, psychiatric, and social consequences of chronic use, but negative effects can be seen even in the short term. Off-hours drinking and substance abuse can contribute to hangovers, withdrawal symptoms, absenteeism, medical and psychiatric complications, and preoccupation with obtaining or using the substances, which can interfere with concentration on the job. Off-duty problems such as charges of driving while intoxicated or drug possession charges are an embarrassment to a company, and legal and illegal off-hours substance abuse can affect employee morale. Use of substances can contribute to corruption and to white-collar crime. Military plane crashes have been found to be associated with use of marijuana, other substances, or alcohol, either by ground crews or flyers. Impairment of physicians is a major problem for the profession, and physicians' health programs have been established in all 50 states. Companies tend to be more punitive for substance abuse than for alcohol. Many companies will require a "Ulysses" contract from substance abusers, which provides that the employees abstain from drugs and that the employer be notified and employment terminated if the employee returns to the habit. Better understanding of prevailing negative attitudes regarding the employee with an SUD and of the particular problems and needs of corporations that employ them will be important. The growing concern of corporate benefits departments requiring cost effectiveness is likely to lead to improvement and sharpening of measurable treatment goals.

Specific Workforce Populations of Concern

There are many work populations. Each may differ in terms of types of drugs used, reasons for use, and potential consequences of use. Results from the National Survey on Drug Use and Health document variations in these areas according to drug use (Figure 14–1) and alcohol use (Figure 14–2).

Athletes

Athletes are usually young adults whose jobs involve a wish for stardom, celebrations, disappointments, access to illicit drugs, large amounts of cash, great physical exertion, and great physiological reserve. Athletes use all kinds of addictive substances recreationally, including cocaine, marijuana, and tobacco. Use may be for enhancement of performance, pleasure, or self-medication of pain. A vast number of substances are used by athletes to improve their performance. Many performance-enhancing drugs have been discovered and regulated; many more exist now, and others will surface in the future. These substances are regulated, mostly because they affect fair competition or because they may endanger the user; these substances include steroids, nutritional supplements, stimulants, or opioids. Professional athletes are role models, and therefore their use of drugs places youth at higher risk than would otherwise be the case. The use of smokeless tobacco is endemic among base-

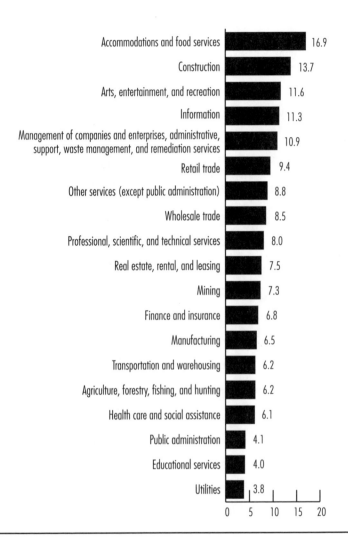

Figure 14–1. Past-month illicit drug use among full-time workers ages 18–64 years, by industry category: 2002–2004 combined.

Source. Substance Abuse and Mental Health Services Administration: The NSDUH Report: Worker Substance Use, by Industry Category. Rockville, MD, Office of Applied Studies, August 23, 2007.

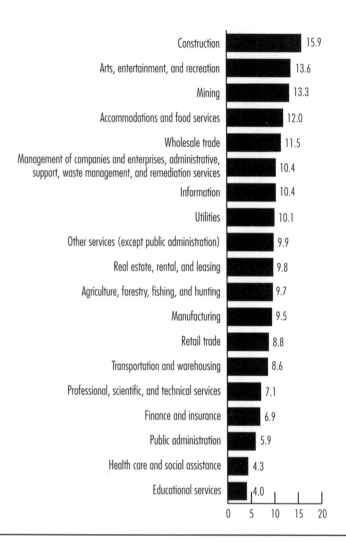

Figure 14–2.   Past-month heavy alcohol use among full-time workers ages 18–64 years, by industry category: 2002–2004 combined.

Source.   Substance Abuse and Mental Health Services Administration: The NSDUH Report: Worker Substance Use, by Industry Category. Rockville, MD, Office of Applied Studies, August 23, 2007.

ball players—even college and high school players (Colborn et al. 1989). Coaches and those concerned about players must be able to make recommendations for treatment regardless of the fame of the player.

Executives and VIPs

Special considerations apply in dealing with substance-abusing leaders, because their impact on other people magnifies the effects of their problems. Moreover, they are often insulated from help by their position, as others fear confronting them. Feeling pressure to appear professional and authoritative, leaders are less likely to seek help or to identify problems. Some have always dealt with emotional distress by covering it over, perhaps through self-medication with drugs or alcohol. Others have relied on the socially lubricating effects of alcohol, or on the short-term performance enhancement of cocaine, for their success. Leaders with addictions feel further impelled to avoid help, and can end up feeling quite "lonely at the top." Yet, being at the top can enable substance use. Executives can make their own schedule in a way that allows for substance use. Some feel that ordinary rules do not apply to them, a feeling that is compounded by the effects of the substance itself. The acquired self-view that accompanies a successful career can lead to difficulty in seeking or accepting help. Awareness of the issues surrounding treatment of the VIP patient and sensitivity to issues related to confidentiality are helpful in treating this category of patients (Martin et al. 2004). There is also a need for the clinician to manage his or her own countertransference in these situations.

Working Youth

Youth in the labor force are at high risk of using substances. A study by the Institute of Medicine (National Research Council and Institute of Medicine 1998) reported the following information:

- High-intensity work (20+ hours per week) is associated with unhealthy behaviors, including substance abuse, insufficient sleep and exercise, and limited time with families.
- The link between intensive work schedules and substance use is found in multiple studies, even after statistical control for background and variables and preexisting conditions such as parental socioeconomic status, race, family composition, and prior substance use.

- Skill utilization (the use of special skills) at work was associated with decreased cigarette and marijuana use. In females, skill utilization was associated with decreased alcohol use.

- Youth who noted that their jobs did not require their skills, and who perceived their jobs to be unconnected to the future, used more cigarettes as the intensity of their work increased.

Health Care Workers

Health care workers are a diverse group, but they share a workplace that combines high stress with some access to addictive substances or to the hardware needed for use. It may be little surprise that substances are often used to cope. All 50 states have systems to monitor physician health and deal with substance abuse in physicians. Abuse is widespread among both nurses and physicians. An anonymous survey (Trinkoff and Storr 1998) revealed that 32% of nurses admitted to use of substances. Physicians may be among the most resistant to seeking help for a real problem despite being at a greater risk than the general population (Aach et al. 1992). Physicians have higher access to pharmaceutical drugs but are less inclined to use street drugs. In the New York State Physicians' Health Program, 88% of the participants used alcohol or prescription drugs and only 12% used marijuana or cocaine. Additional risk for SUDs in physicians have been postulated to be "pharmacological optimism," intellectual strength, strong will, love of challenges, instrumental use of medications, and a daily need for denial (Mansky 1999). As in other professions, there may be a need to tailor treatments for this group, especially to protect their confidentiality.

High-Responsibility Workers

High-responsibility workers include air traffic personnel, machine operators, drivers, and pilots. For the worker with people's lives in his or her hands, there may be no "safe" level of blood alcohol. One British study demonstrated that, despite a lack of sense of sleepiness, drivers driving during the typical "circadian dip" following a lunch with alcohol who were at half the legal limit nonetheless performed worse on driving and had altered electroencephalographies (EEGs) (Horne et al. 2003). Blood alcohol levels as low as 0.04% may be sufficient to impair one's ability to pilot a plane (Dave 2004). It is important to not ignore the effects of nicotine: pilots may go through nicotine withdrawal during flight (Giannakoulas et al. 2003). The American Society of Addiction Medicine guidelines (Mee-Lee et al. 2001) recognize that reporting substance abuse is necessary when there is an "immediate threat to public safety."

The danger is not just limited to flying and driving. A study of railroad occupational accident investigations revealed that positive test findings were more common in fatal than nonfatal accidents. In approximately one-third of the accidents associated with positive drug test results, alcohol and/or drug use was determined to be related to accident causation (National Institute on Drug Abuse 1990).

Police/Military

Police and military workers may be at high risk of harm when intoxicated, in that they have access to lethal weapons. There are countless anecdotes about suicides and murders committed by policemen while intoxicated. Those who learn to kill during war may be more prone not just to substance use, but also to violence and posttraumatic stress disorder (PTSD), with signs of these apparent in the workplace. In the armed forces, performance-enhancing drugs may be more prevalent than recreational ones. There is anecdotal evidence that military pilots are increasingly being asked to use sedatives for sleep and stimulants during the period of their missions (Shanker and Duenwald 2003). This may lead to more public concern and inquiry.

Public Policy on Prevention and Control

Role of Prevention

With greater scientific advances in understanding of alcoholism and other addictions in terms of description, etiology, pathogenesis, course, and epidemiology, there is an increasing possibility that strategies for prevention may be successful. Advances in genetic understanding of familial alcoholism, for example, may lead to discovery of markers that can identify a high-risk population. However, we are still far from being able to match prevention of infectious disease by vaccination and prevention of parasitic disease by improved sanitary and public health measures. Efforts at border control, increased public information, and improved efforts at social planning in law enforcement have not led to major changes in the magnitude of the problem.

The vast cost of the problem requires greater research, so that a better understanding of the illness, its prevention, and its treatment may be developed.

Mass Media Campaigns

Mass media prevention campaigns via radio, television, and print use popular peer models as well as messages delivered by prominent sports figures, celebrities, or parental role models. An active public service announcement campaign of donated advertising time produced by Partnership for a Drug-Free America (which has been supplemented with federal financing) has been very effective in changing attitudes, challenging myths, and promoting increased communication between parents and children about drugs. Between 1997 and 1999, illicit substance use among adolescents (ages 12–17 years) significantly declined, perhaps as a result of this program. This effort in part counters advertisers' use of mass media to increase sales of addictive substances (e.g., alcohol, tobacco). Use and abuse of psychoactive substances are frequently glamorized on television and in films. Commercials that portray alcohol use in a positive light, with images of camaraderie, relaxation, and enjoyment, contain important subliminal messages, although it is not clear whether and to what extent such advertising negatively impacts prevention efforts. Alcohol-containing products such as wine coolers, frequently packaged to look like soft drinks, are sold over the counter in grocery stores and are designed to appeal to a youth market.

Social Policy and Legal Efforts

Greater availability of addictive substances leads to greater craving for them and higher use. Because alcohol and tobacco are widely available, cheap, and legal, they are the most heavily used. Due to the enormous profits that can be gleaned from the sale of drugs, it has proved to be extremely difficult to limit the influx of illegal substances. Illegal drug use is tied to market value, cost, availability, and quality. Limiting availability of alcohol through price manipulation, outlet availability, hours of sale, and age restriction policies is one strategy to reduce overall consumption. Forbidding grocery stores from selling distilled alcohol and the banning of hotel room refrigerated beverage dispensers are examples of efforts to reduce exposure of recovering alcoholics and teenagers to marketing pressures that increase availability. Overall rates of liver cirrhosis are correlated with alcohol availability and total alcohol consumption, and may be reduced by efforts to limit consumption. The legal drinking age has been raised to 21 years throughout the nation, and studies indicate that this has decreased motor vehicle accidents and deaths among adolescents. Unfortunately, too little effort has been put into enforcing this limit on college campuses, where binge drinking has become endemic. Limiting tobacco advertising and use in public places has been another effective measure in an effort to achieve the Surgeon General's goal of a "smokeless" society (U.S. Department of Health and Human Services 2000). In addition to governmental agreements with tobacco companies, private litigation has led to large settlements or awards, and more of those assets should be used to further public health efforts. Of note, there is good reason to believe that schizophrenic patients can successfully tolerate smoking cessation programs (Addington et al. 1998).

Public Sector Clinical Approaches

High-Risk Populations

Children of Alcoholics

Twin, adoption, and half-sibling genetic studies and studies of familial versus nonfamilial alcoholism indicate that children of alcoholics are at fourfold higher risk of developing alcoholism. Fifty percent to 70% of the variance of addiction to substances has been attributed to genetics (Kendler and Prescott 1998). Efforts to target programs for those at high risk for heart disease, obesity, hypertension, and high cholesterol have been paralleled by programs to assist the high-risk group of children of alcoholics in achieving alternative alcohol-free lifestyles. Familial alcoholics have an earlier onset of problem drinking, more severe social consequences, less consistently stable family involvement, poorer academic and social performance in school, more antisocial behavior, and poorer prognosis in treatment.

A major movement has grown up around the problem of being an adult child of an alcoholic. As children, these individuals frequently suffer from stigma, alienation, estrangement, and isolation. Their parents are frequently inconsistent and emotionally depriving, force them into inappropriate roles, are more likely to be aggressive or sexually abusing, and are more likely to have difficult divorces and may abandon their children. Struggling with feelings of anger, confusion, and helplessness, these children tend to distrust authority figures, depend more on peers, and pick friends from similarly troubled families. Distrust of authority figures is likely to extend to doctors, nurses, and other health care professionals. These children grow up protesting their parents' behavior, trying to be different, but ending up with the same problems. This may explain why self-help groups, group therapy, and family approaches that take into account peer support are so successful.

College Students

Despite continued efforts to reduce abuse of alcohol among teens and college students, problems continue; binge drinking is rampant on college campuses as well as in high school settings. Freshmen, who are often away from home for the first time, may perceive drinking and substance experimentation as "cool" and as an entry into a fraternity or sorority, some of which may foster heavy drinking. One study showed that brief intervention as a primary step might be helpful especially if done in a nonjudgmental, practical way (Marlatt et al. 1998). Lack of supervision of students by universities and colleges contributes to the problem. Most colleges have inadequate programs for alcohol abuse prevention, detection, and treatment. Designated driver programs are helpful in harm reduction.

Reducing the availability of cheap alcohol to underage students would help. A major change in the cultural trend and efforts to reduce social supports for drinking on college campuses are needed. Concerned parents must hold college administrators accountable to enforce rules regulating alcohol use on campuses and should encourage colleges to provide safe housing for recovering students and student counseling services regarding addiction. Some colleges have taken a lead in developing programs to help students in recovery by providing sober dorms, counseling, and peer leaders. Parents with children at risk should consider these issues in choosing the right school for their children.

Relationship of Substance Abuse Treatment to Other Public Prevention Efforts

Early treatment of an alcohol or drug problem may also help prevent development of other problems, such as depression or antisocial personality. Similarly, early treatment of depression, attention-deficit/hyperactivity disorder, or anxiety disorders may help to prevent the development of an alcohol or drug problem, and thereby progression to antisocial personality. These illnesses have complicated interactions, and each can precede, contribute to, or coexist with the others. Attention-deficit/hyperactivity disorder can be seen as a "gateway disorder" in which there should be early identification and intervention of SUDs.

Attempts at preventing tuberculosis and human immunodeficiency virus (HIV), which are often comorbid with substance misuse, have diverged. HIV is finally at a plateau of new cases, but tuberculosis remains rampant. With multidrug-resistant tuberculosis, it is all the more important to develop a systematic services approach to protect caregivers and patients alike (Perlman et al. 1995). For HIV in the United States, however, the story has recently taken a positive turn (Des Jarlais et al. 2000). The need for patient education and treatment and heightened awareness of risks is great.

Public Trauma

The experiences of September 11, 2001 (Vlahov et al. 2004), and of war in other nations have documented that even in the absence of PTSD, there is an increase in use of substances. For Israeli youth closely exposed to violence, for example, there have been temporary increases in use of alcohol and cannabis, although not cigarettes (Schiff et al. 2007). This has been shown in both military and civilian populations, with women suffering more psychopathology as a result (Greiger et al. 2003). Alcohol use increased among victims of the 1995 Oklahoma City bombing. This increase was not generally successful in alleviating symptoms, but rather was associated with increased functional impairment. Use of substances increases vulnerability to PTSD (Pfefferbaum and Doughty 2001).

Public sector services for mental health are more often than not separated from substance use agencies and channels. This separation has seemed artificial, and the result leads to insufficient cross-training and poor collaboration and referral from one system to another. Patients need integrated care, and systems making this happen are at the cutting edge (Havassy et al. 2004).

Key Points

- The workplace is a venue that is affected by the negative consequences of substance abuse, and can potentially be a place where people at risk can be identified early and treated through programs such as employee assistance programs.

- Efforts at identifying and reducing substance abuse can be tailored to specific populations such as pilots, health care workers, and adolescents through understanding the unique attributes and needs of the population.

- The problem is great enough that efforts to prevent substance abuse have to be focused on both the general public as well as the workplace.

References

Aach RD, Girard DE, Humphrey H, et al: Alcohol and other substance abuse and impairment among physicians in residency training. Ann Intern Med 116:245–254, 1992

Addington J, el-Guebaly N, Campbell W, et al: Smoking cessation treatment for patients with schizophrenia. Am J Psychiatry155:974–976, 1998

Bachman JG, Wallace JM Jr, O'Malley PM: Racial/ethnic differences in smoking, drinking, and illicit drug use among American high school seniors, 1976–1989. Am J Public Health 81:372–377, 1991

Blum TC, Martin JK, Roman PM: A research note of EAP prevalence, components, and utilization. Journal of Employee Assistance Research 1:209–229, 1992

Colborn JW, Cummings KM, Michaelek AM: Correlates of adolescents' use of smokeless tobacco. Health Ed Q 16:91–100, 1989

Dave BP: Flying under the influence of alcohol. J Clin Forensic Med 11:12–14, 2004

Des Jarlais DC, Marmor M, Friedmann P, et al: HIV incidence among injection drug users in New York City, 1992–1997: evidence for a declining epidemic. Am J Public Health 90:352–359, 2000

Giannakoulas G, Katramados A, Melas N, et al: Acute effects of nicotine withdrawal syndrome in pilots during flight. Aviat Space Environ Med 74:247–251, 2003

Greiger TA, Fullerton CS, Ursano RJ: Posttraumatic stress disorder, alcohol use, and perceived safety after the terrorist attack on the Pentagon. Psychiatr Serv 54:1380–1382, 2003

Havassy BE, Alvidrez J, Owen KK: Comparisons of patients with comorbid psychiatric and substance use disorders: implications for treatment and service delivery. Am J Psychiatry 161:139–145, 2004

Horne JA, Reyner LA, Barrett PR: Driving impairment due to sleepiness is exacerbated by low alcohol intake. Occup Environ Med 60:689–692, 2003

Kendler KS, Prescott CA: Cocaine use, abuse, and dependence in a population-based sample of female twins. Br J Psychiatry 173:345–350, 1998

Mansky PA: Issues in the recovery of physicians from addictive illnesses. Psychiatr Q 70:107–122, 1999

Marlatt GA, Baer JS, Kivlahan DR, et al: Screening and brief intervention for high-risk college student drinkers: results from a 2-year follow-up assessment. J Consult Clin Psychol 66:604–615, 1998

Martin A, Bostic J, Pruett K: The V.I.P.: hazard and promise in treating "special" patients. J Am Acad Child Adolesc Psychiatry 43:366–369, 2004

Mee-Lee D, Shulman GR, Fishman M, et al: ASAM PPC-2R: American Society of Addiction Medicine Patient Placement Criteria for the Treatment of Substance-Related Disorders, 2nd Edition—Revised. Chevy Chase, MD, American Society of Addiction Medicine, 2001

Merrick ES, Volpe-Vartanian J, Horgan CM, et al: Alcohol and drug use: revisiting employee assistance programs and substance use problems in the workplace: key issues and a research agenda. Psychiatr Serv 58:1262–1264, 2007

National Institute on Alcohol Abuse and Alcoholism: Alcohol Alert 44. July 1999. Available at: http://pubs.niaaa.nih.gov/publications/aa44.htm. Accessed June 20, 2009.

National Institute on Alcohol Abuse and Alcoholism: Alcohol Alert 51. January 2001. Available at: http://pubs.niaaa.nih.gov/publications/aa51.htm. Accessed June 20, 2009.

National Institute on Drug Abuse: Drugs in the workplace: research and evaluation data, NIDA Res Monogr 100:3–238, 1990. Available at: www.nida.nih.gov/pdf/monographs/download100.html. Accessed June 20, 2009.

National Research Council and Institute of Medicine, Committee on the Health and Safety Implications of Child Labor. Protecting Youth at Work: Health, Safety, and Development of Working Children and Adolescents in the United States. Washington, DC, National Academies Press, 1998

Office of National Drug Control Policy: The Economic Costs of Drug Abuse in the United States, 1992–1998 (Publ No NCJ-190636). Washington, DC, Executive Office of the President, 2001

Open Minds: Yearbook of Managed Behavioral Health and Employee Assistance Program Market Share in the United States, 2002–2003. Gettysburg, PA, OPEN MINDS, October 2002. Available at: www.openminds.com/pressroom/mbhoyearbook02.htm. Accessed June 20, 2009.

Perlman DC, Saloman N, Perkins MP, et al: Tuberculosis in drug users. Clin Infect Dis 21:1263–1264, 1995

Pfefferbaum B, Doughty DE: Increased alcohol use in a treatment sample of Oklahoma City bombing victims. Psychiatry 64:296–303, 2001

Schiff M Zweig HH, Benbenishty R, et al: Exposure to terrorism and Israeli youths' cigarette, alcohol, and cannabis use. Am J Public Health 97:1852–1858, 2007

Shanker T, Duenwald M: Threats and responses: military, bombing error puts a spotlight on pilots' pills. New York Times, January 19, 2003

Substance Abuse and Mental Health Services Administration: Results From the 2006 National Survey on Drug Use and Health: National Findings (NSDUH Series H-32; DHHS Publ No SMA 07-4293). Rockville, MD, Office of Applied Studies, 2007

Trinkoff AM, Storr CL: Substance use among nurses: differences among specialties. Am J Public Health 88:581–555, 1998

U.S. Department of Health and Human Services: Reducing Tobacco Use: A Report of the Surgeon General. Atlanta, GA, Centers for Disease Control and Prevention, National Center for Chronic Disease Prevention and Health Promotion, Office on Smoking and Health, 2000

Vlahov D, Galea S Ahern J: Sustained increased consumption of cigarettes, alcohol, and marijuana among Manhattan residents after September 11, 2001. Am J Public Health 94:253–254, 2004

Appendix: Workplace Substance Abuse Resources

- National Partnership for Workplace Mental Health (http://www.workplacementalhealth.org)
- National Clearinghouse for Alcohol and Drug Information: Workplace (http://ncadi.samhsa.gov/features/workplace)
- Parents: The Anti-Drug (http://www.theantidrug.com)
- Substance Abuse and Mental Health Services Administration: Division of Workplace Programs (http://www.workplace.samhsa.gov)
- White House Office of National Drug Control Policy (ONDCP): Drug-Free Workplace (www.whitehousedrugpolicy.gov/prevent/workplace/index.html)

Index

*Page numbers printed in **boldface** type refer to tables or figures.*